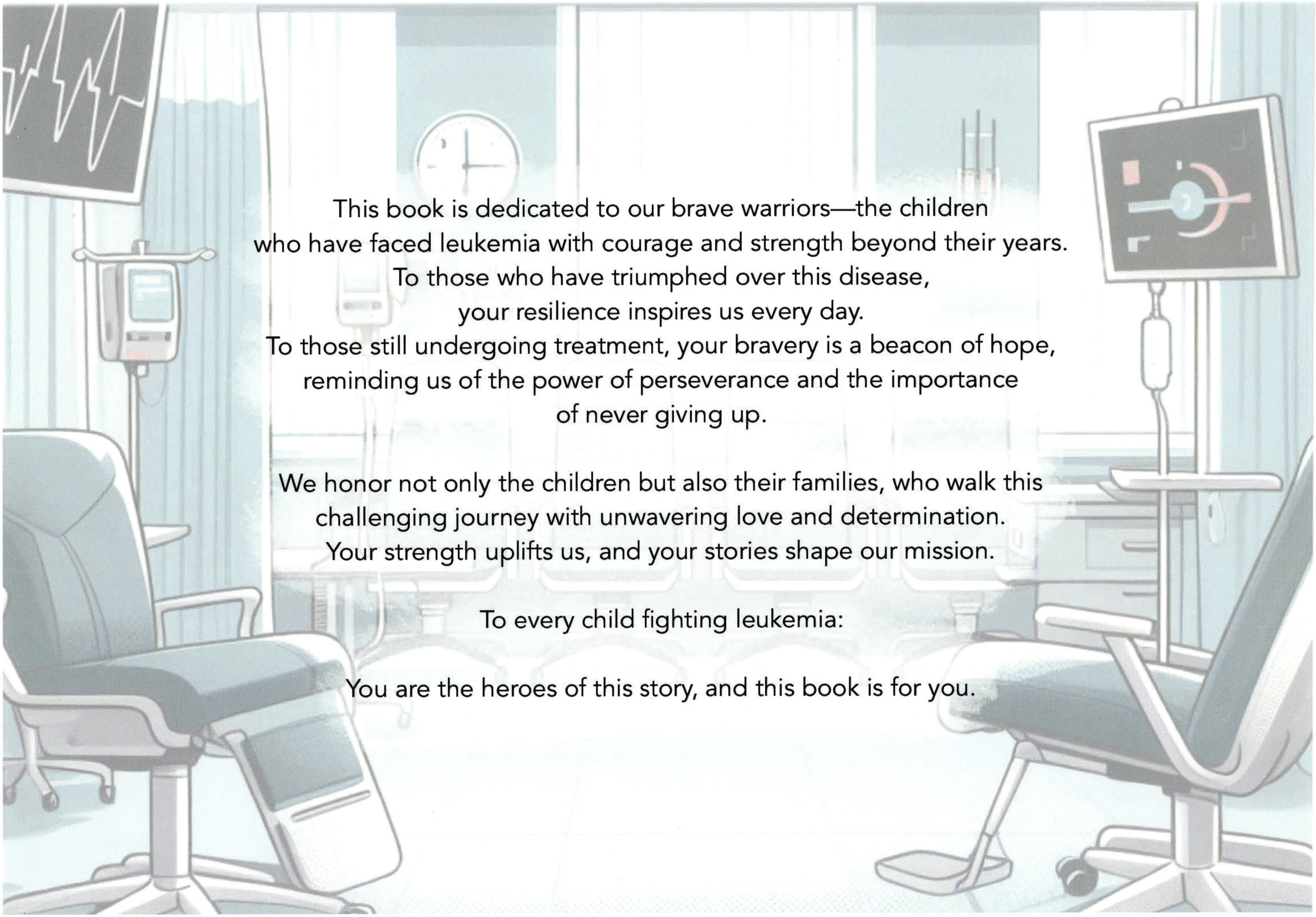

This book is dedicated to our brave warriors—the children
who have faced leukemia with courage and strength beyond their years.
To those who have triumphed over this disease,
your resilience inspires us every day.
To those still undergoing treatment, your bravery is a beacon of hope,
reminding us of the power of perseverance and the importance
of never giving up.

We honor not only the children but also their families, who walk this
challenging journey with unwavering love and determination.
Your strength uplifts us, and your stories shape our mission.

To every child fighting leukemia:

You are the heroes of this story, and this book is for you.

Allison's Adventure

This is a story of a brave young girl who faces leukemia, who sees her struggle as a battle within her own body. With the love and support of her family, doctors, and friends, she triumphs over cancer.

Dr Krista Francisco, author and illustrator
Senior Resident Physician
Division of Paediatric Haematology/Oncology/BMT
Khoo Teck Puat-National University Children's Medical Institute, NUHS

Noorleeyahti Binte Ramjudi, co-author and illustrator
Assistant Nurse Clinician/Clinical Instructor, Ward 8B
Division of Paediatric Haematology/Oncology/BMT
Khoo Teck Puat-National University Children's Medical Institute, NUHS

Professor Allen Yeoh, editor
VIVA-Goh Foundation Professor in Paediatric Oncology, NUS
Head, Division of Paediatric Haematology/Oncology/BMT
Khoo Teck Puat-National University Children's Medical Institute, NUHS

KTP-NUCMI is a part of the National University Centre for Women and Children (NUWoC)

ISBN 978-981-9812-37-0
This book is supported by an educational or charitable donation from AMGEN.
Printed in Singapore

AMGEN

NUS National University of Singapore | Department of Paediatrics
Yong Loo Lin School of Medicine

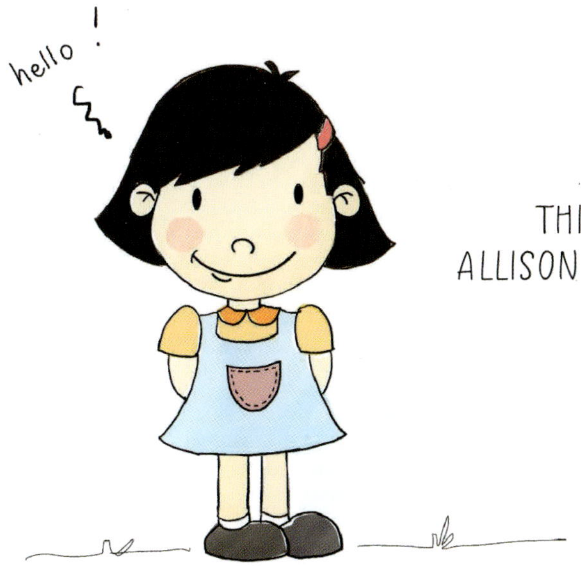

THIS IS ALLISON.
ALLISON IS A HAPPY GIRL.

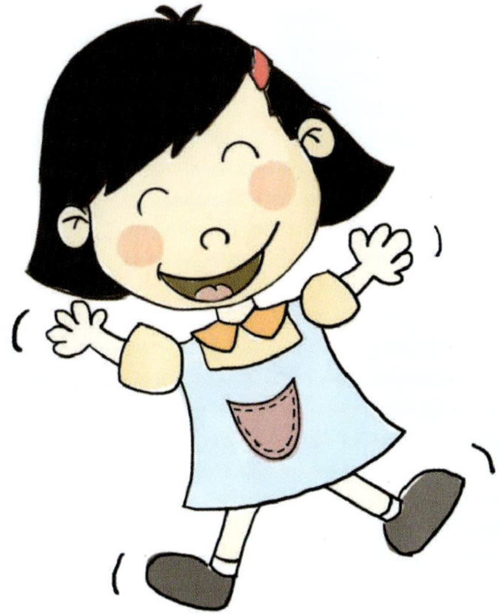

SHE LIKES DANCING
AND PLAYING.

AND GOING TO SCHOOL!

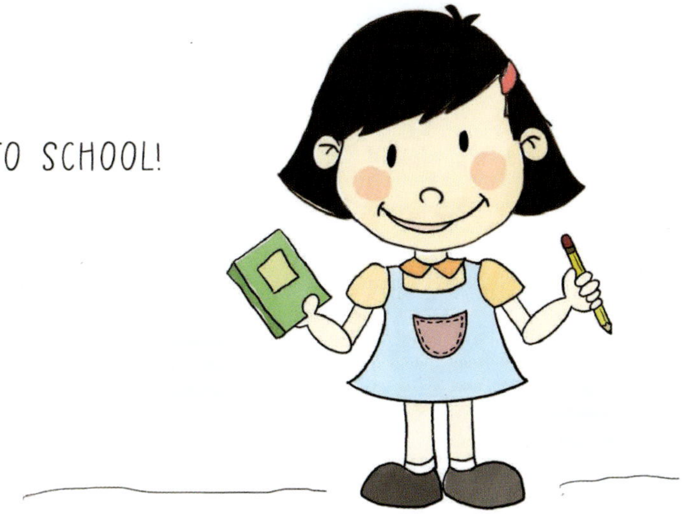

ONE DAY, ALLISON HAD A FEVER.
SHE DID NOT FEEL WELL.

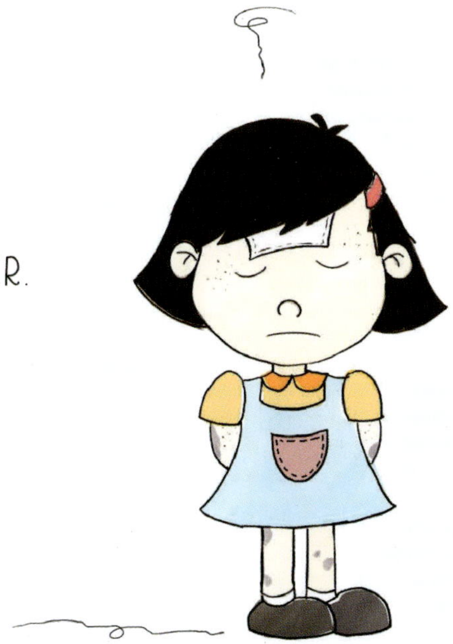

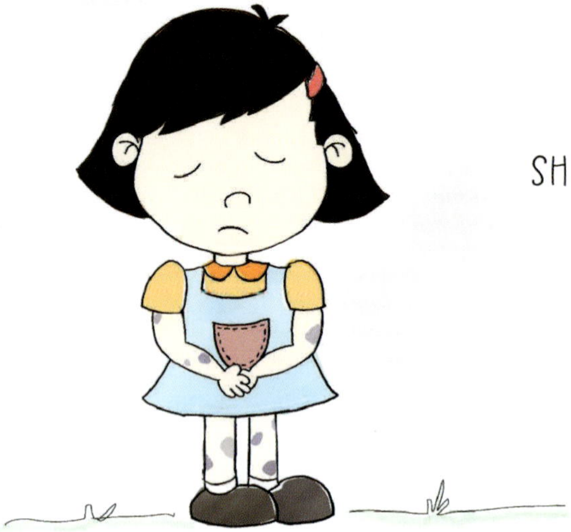

SHE HAD BIG BLUE SPOTS...

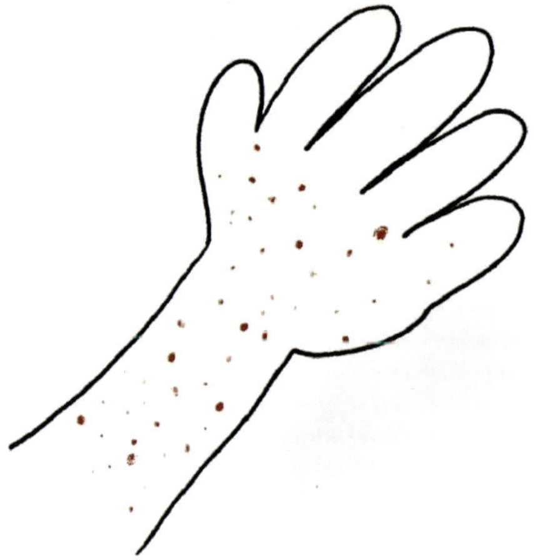

AND SMALL RED DOTS
ALL OVER.

THERE WAS BLOOD FROM HER
NOSE AND ON HER
TOOTHBRUSH TOO.
IT WAS SO SCARY!

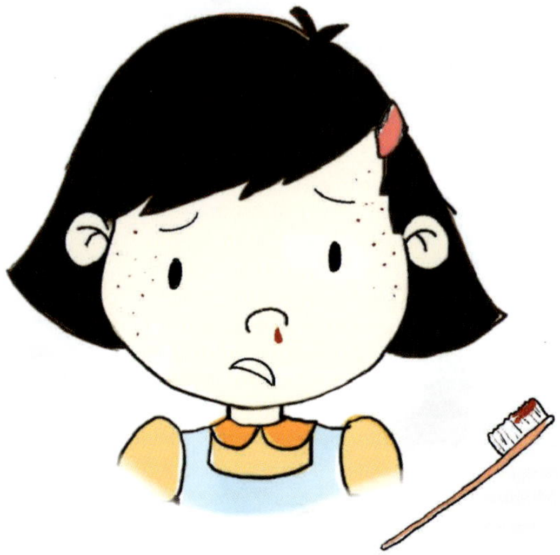

ALLISON WAS ALWAYS TIRED
AND SHE DID NOT WANT
TO PLAY ANYMORE.

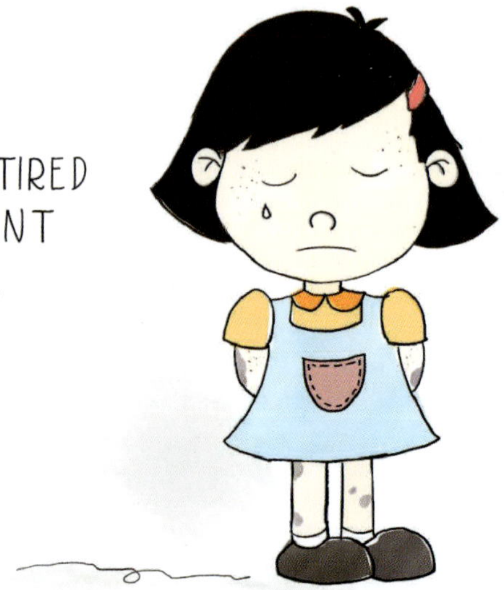

ALLISON'S MOM AND DAD WERE VERY WORRIED SO THEY BROUGHT HER HOME FROM SCHOOL.

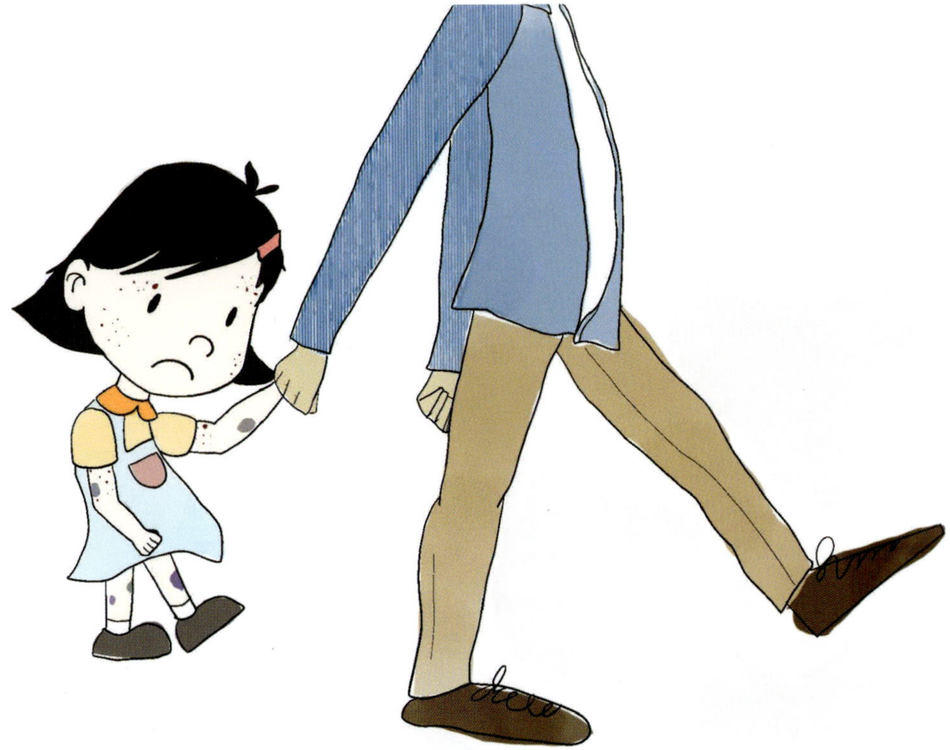

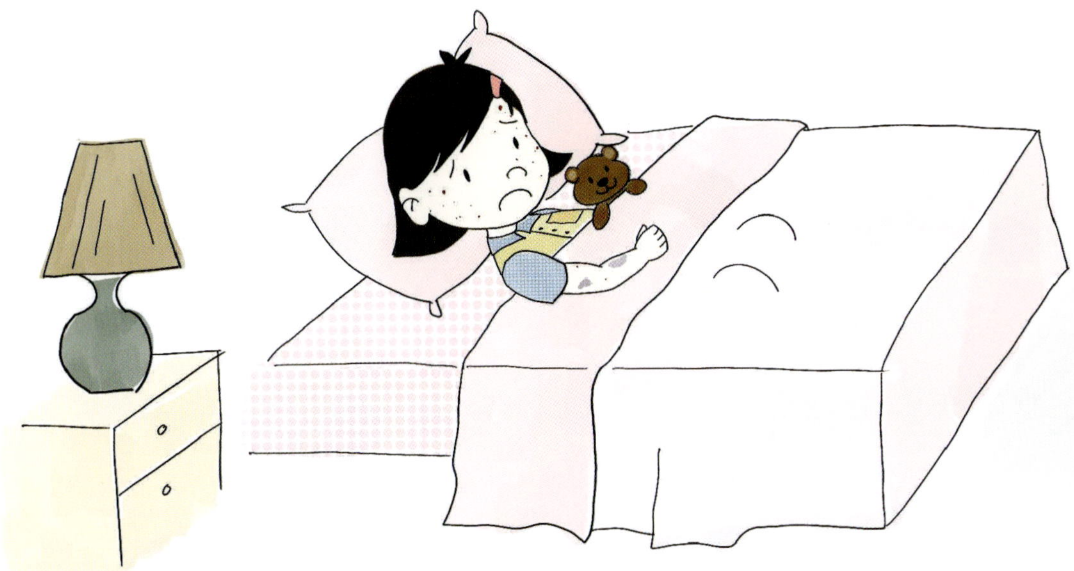

"ALLISON, WE'RE GOING TO THE DOCTOR TOMORROW," HER MOM SAID.

THAT NIGHT, ALLISON COULD NOT SLEEP...

AND WHEN SHE DID,

SHE HAD A VERY STRANGE DREAM.

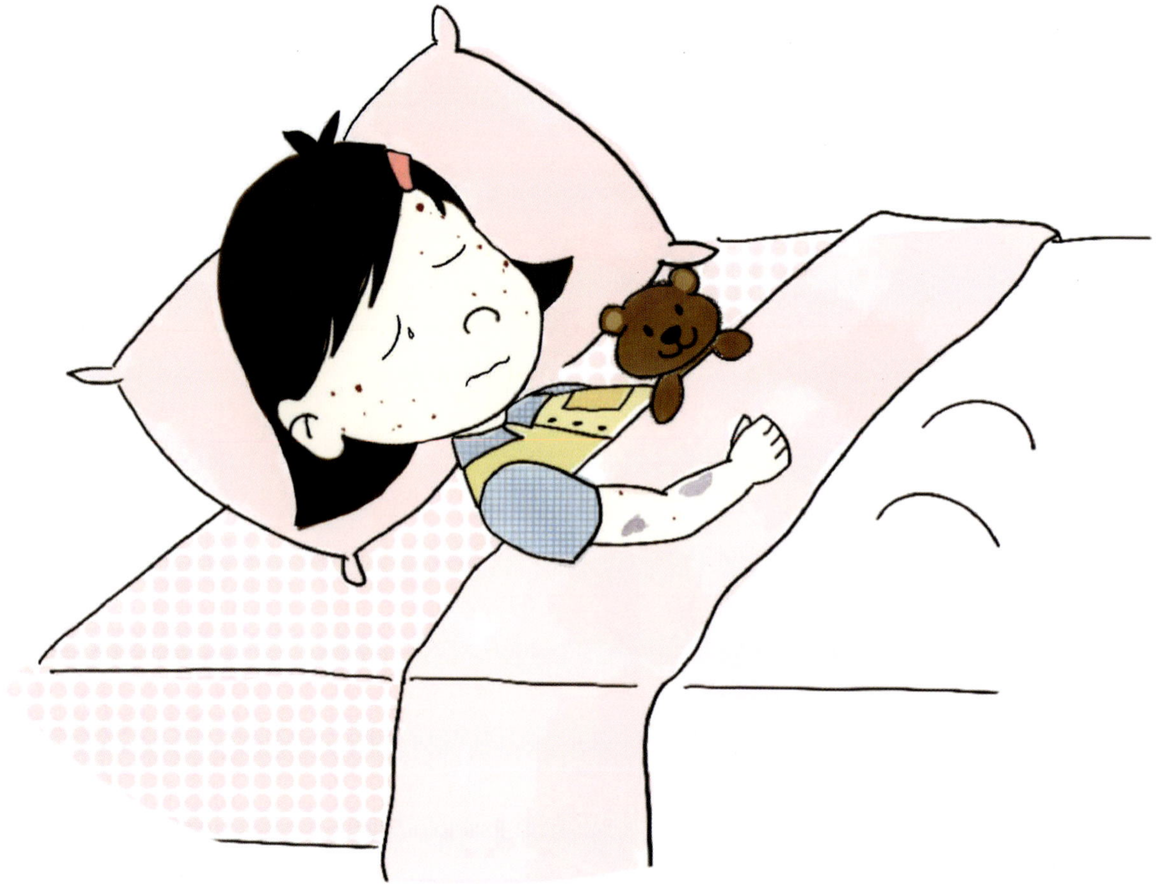

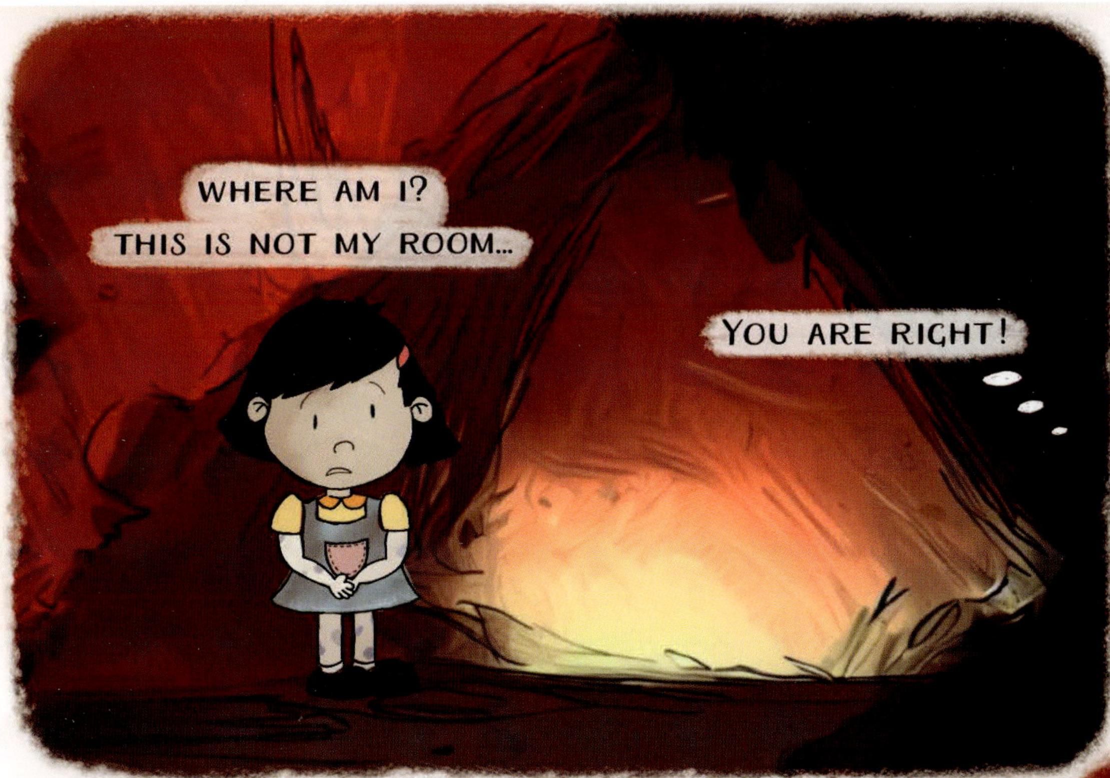
WHERE AM I?
THIS IS NOT MY ROOM...
YOU ARE RIGHT!

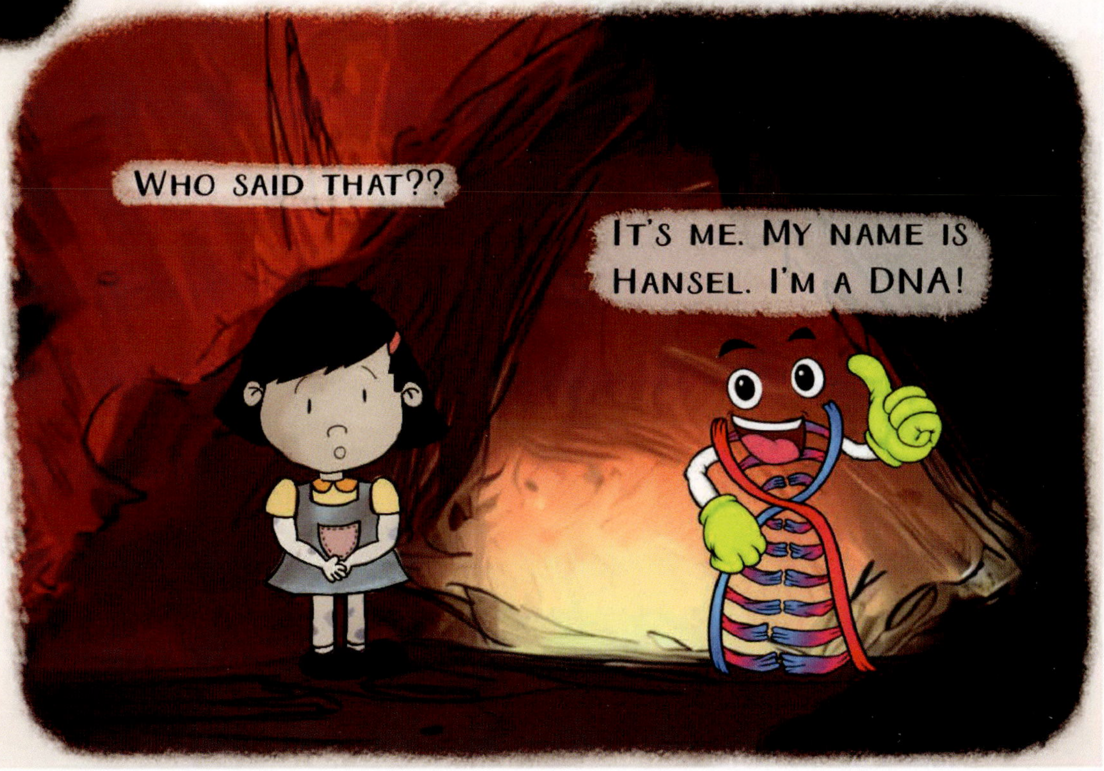
WHO SAID THAT??
IT'S ME. MY NAME IS HANSEL. I'M A DNA!

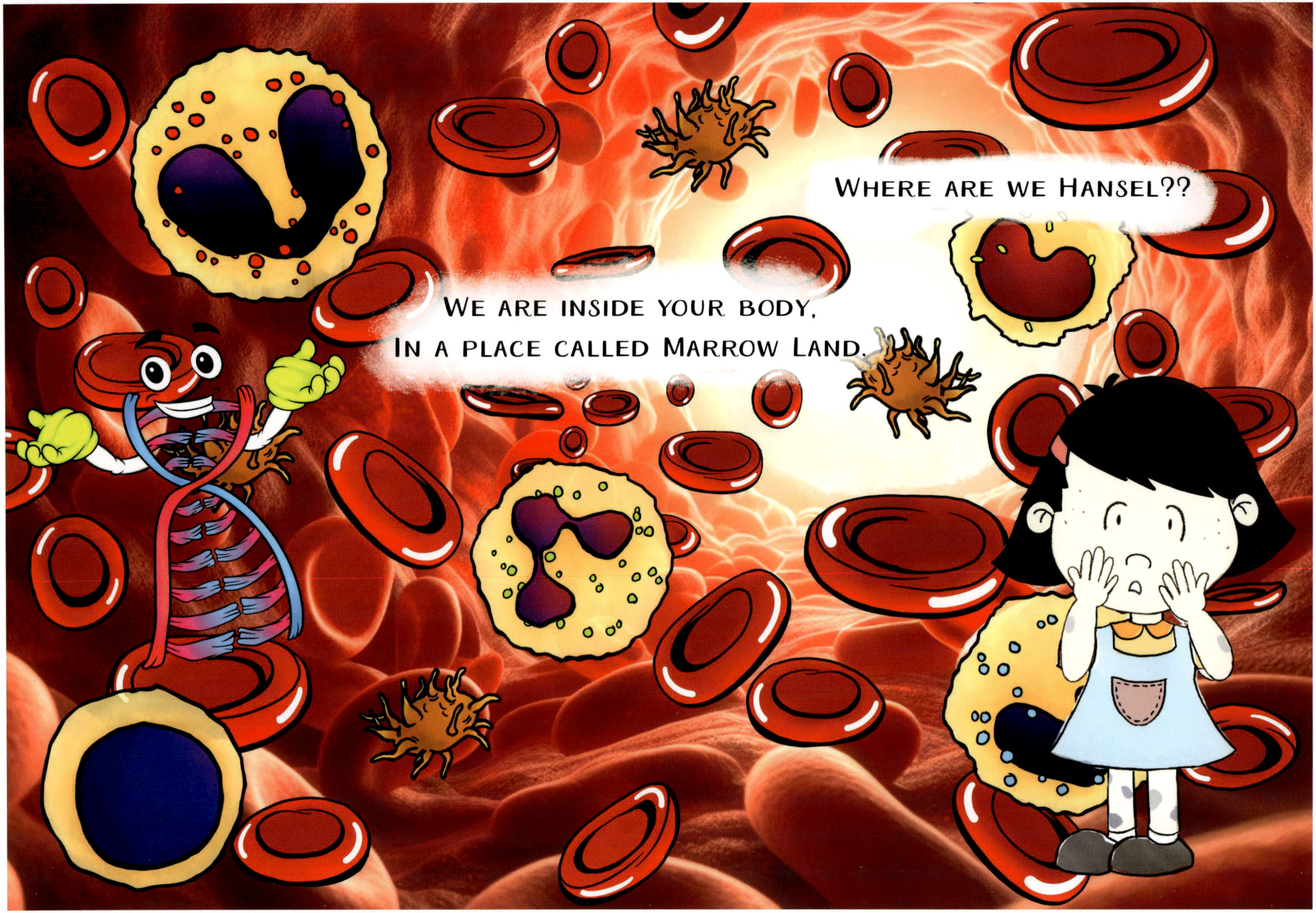
WHERE ARE WE HANSEL??
WE ARE INSIDE YOUR BODY,
IN A PLACE CALLED MARROW LAND.

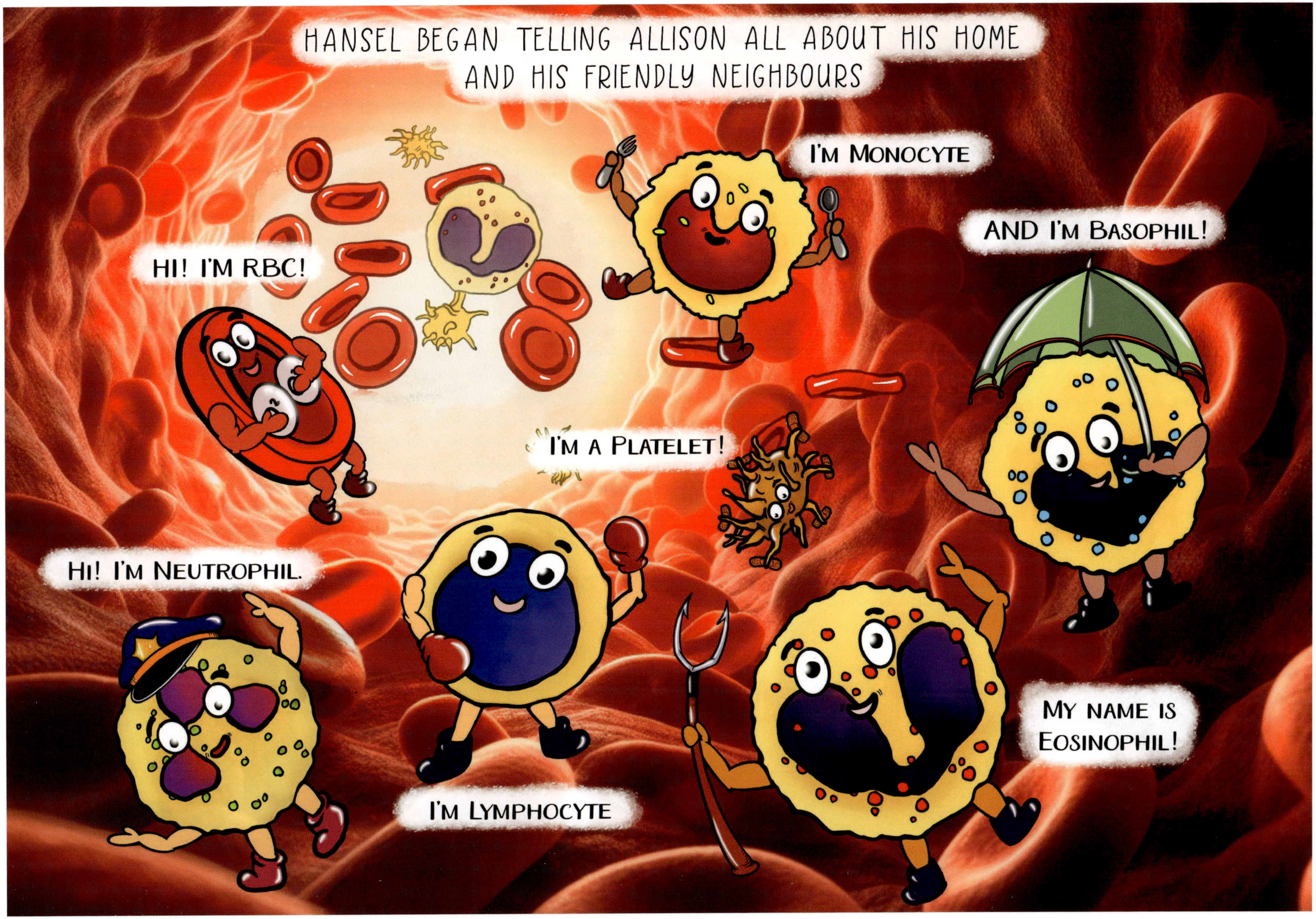
HANSEL BEGAN TELLING ALLISON ALL ABOUT HIS HOME AND HIS FRIENDLY NEIGHBOURS
HI! I'M RBC!
I'M MONOCYTE
AND I'M BASOPHIL!
I'M A PLATELET!
HI! I'M NEUTROPHIL.
I'M LYMPHOCYTE
MY NAME IS EOSINOPHIL!

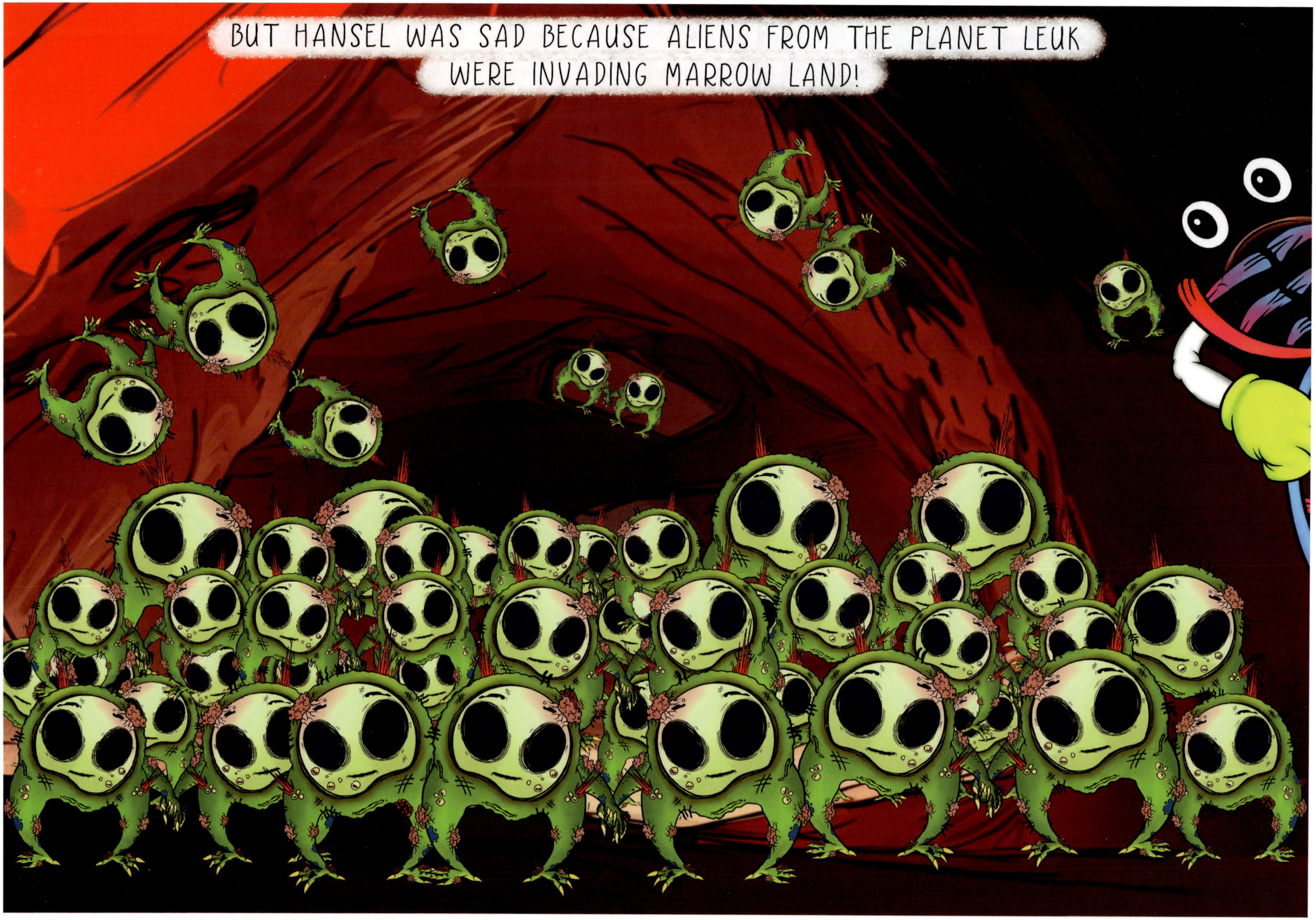
BUT HANSEL WAS SAD BECAUSE ALIENS FROM THE PLANET LEUK WERE INVADING MARROW LAND!

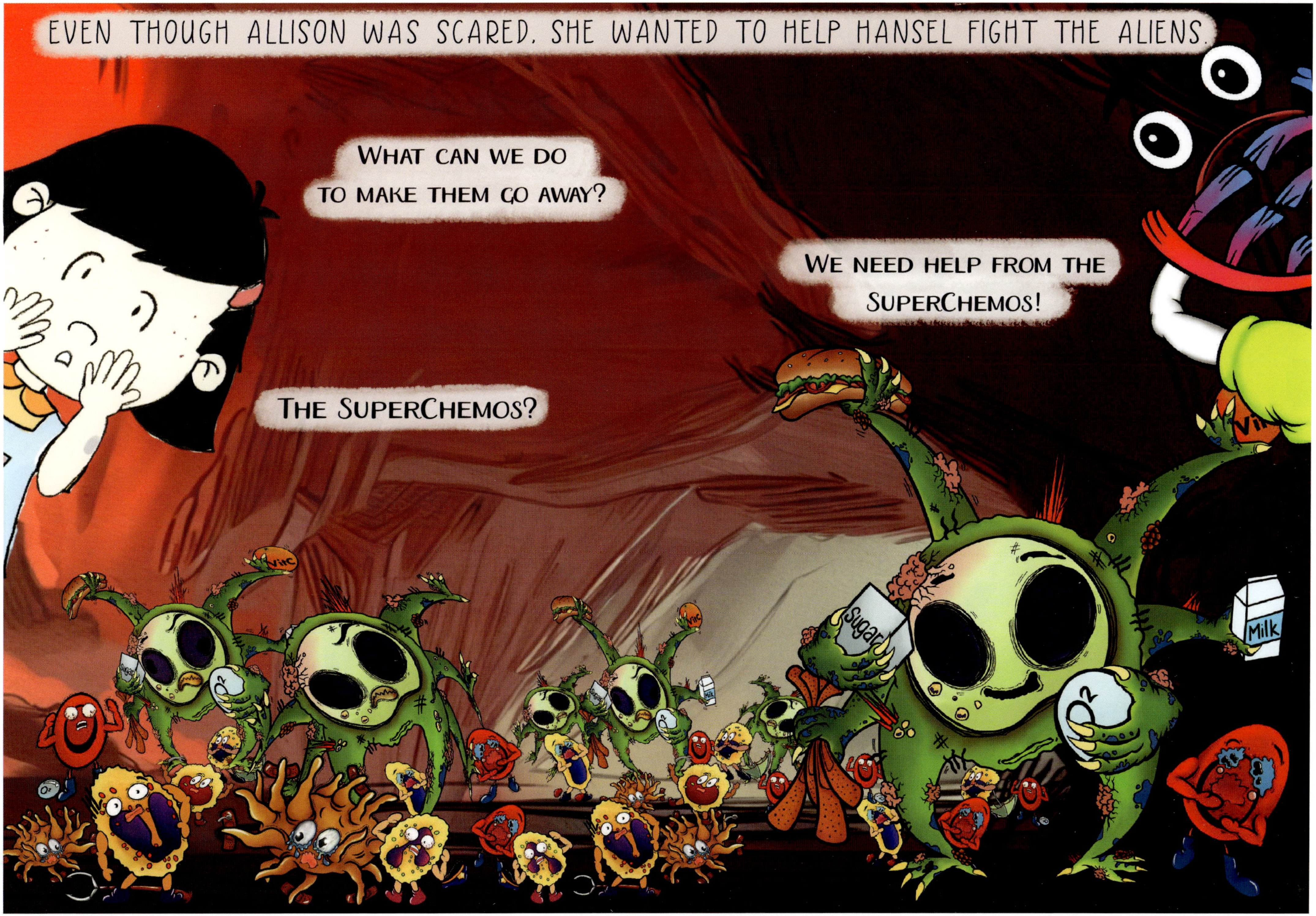
EVEN THOUGH ALLISON WAS SCARED, SHE WANTED TO HELP HANSEL FIGHT THE ALIENS.
WHAT CAN WE DO TO MAKE THEM GO AWAY?
WE NEED HELP FROM THE SUPERCHEMOS!
THE SUPERCHEMOS?
Sugar
Milk

BUT BEFORE HANSEL COULD ANSWER, ALLISON WOKE UP BACK IN HER ROOM.

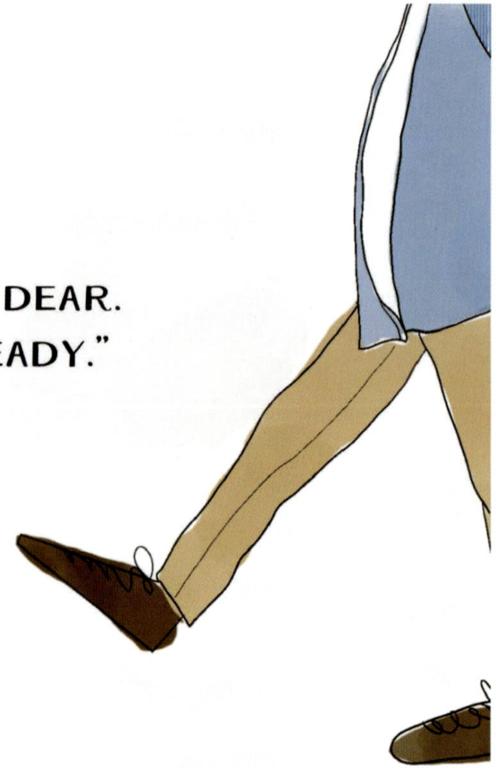

"ALLISON? WAKE UP DEAR.
IT'S TIME TO GET READY."

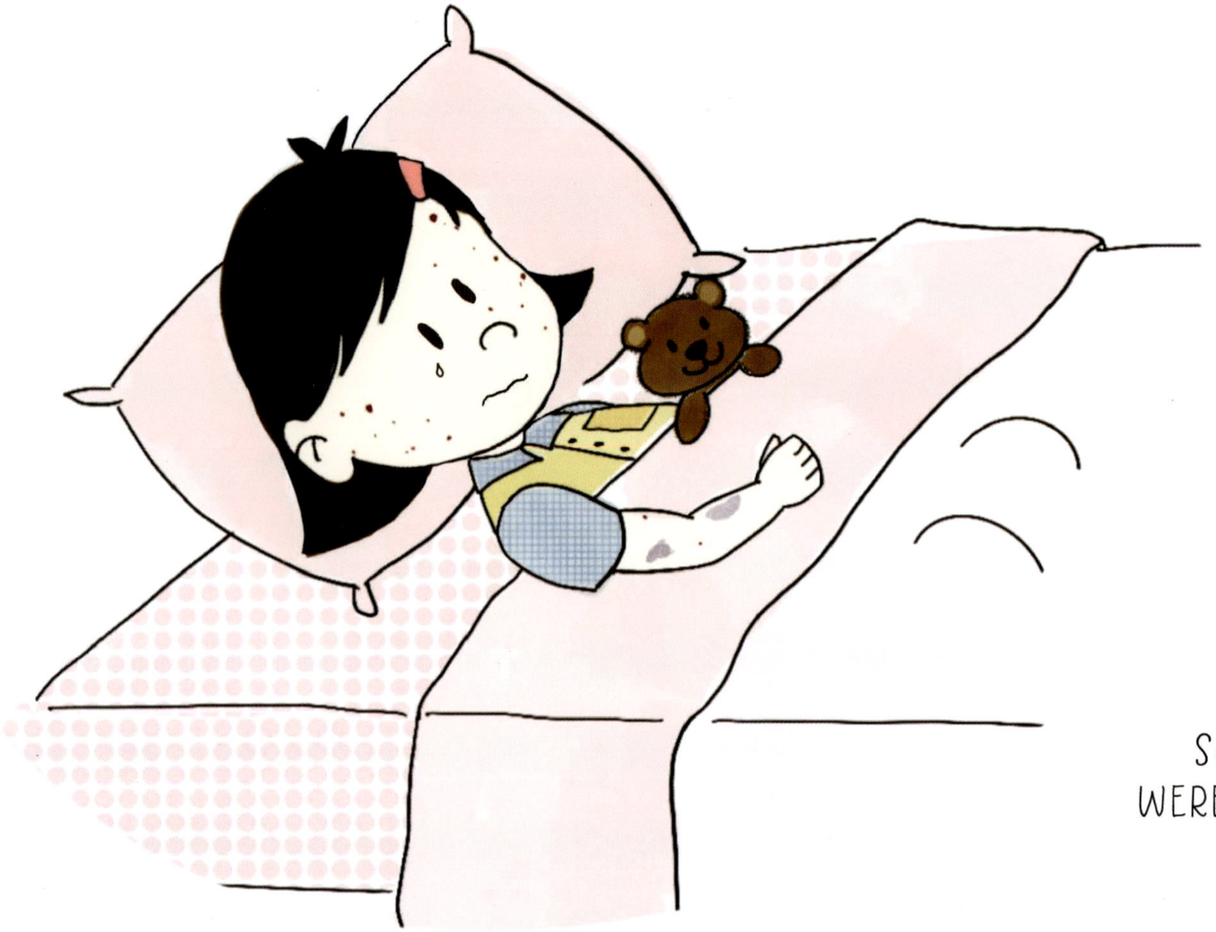

SOON, ALLISON AND HER PARENTS
WERE ON THEIR WAY TO THE HOSPITAL.

ALLISON SAT QUIETLY IN HER CHAIR
BECAUSE SHE WAS SHY AND SCARED.

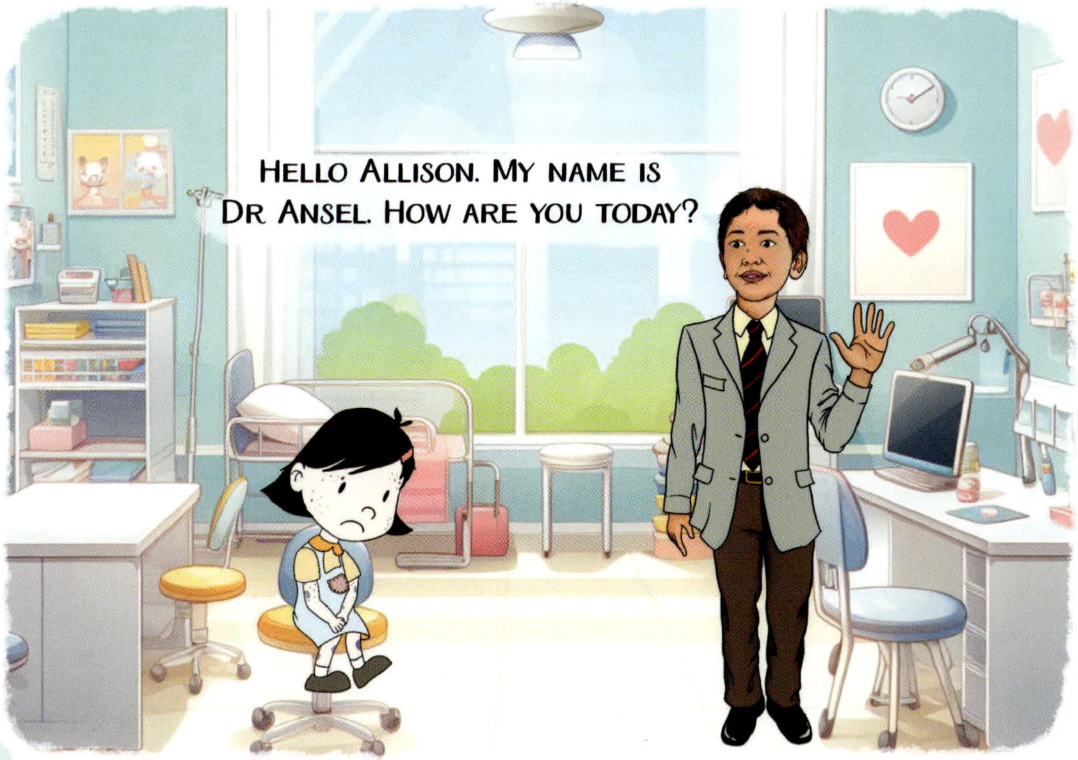
HELLO ALLISON. MY NAME IS
DR ANSEL. HOW ARE YOU TODAY?

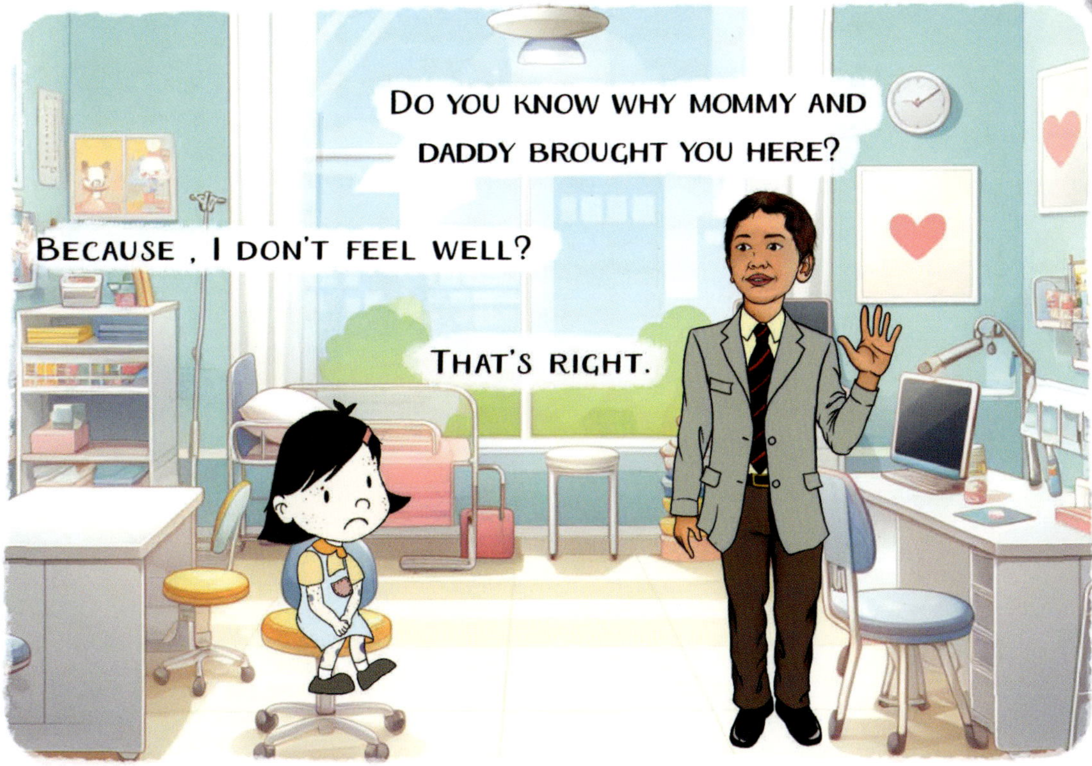
DO YOU KNOW WHY MOMMY AND
DADDY BROUGHT YOU HERE?
BECAUSE , I DON'T FEEL WELL?
THAT'S RIGHT.

THE DOCTOR SEEMED ODDLY FAMILIAR...
HE SOUNDED JUST LIKE HANSEL!

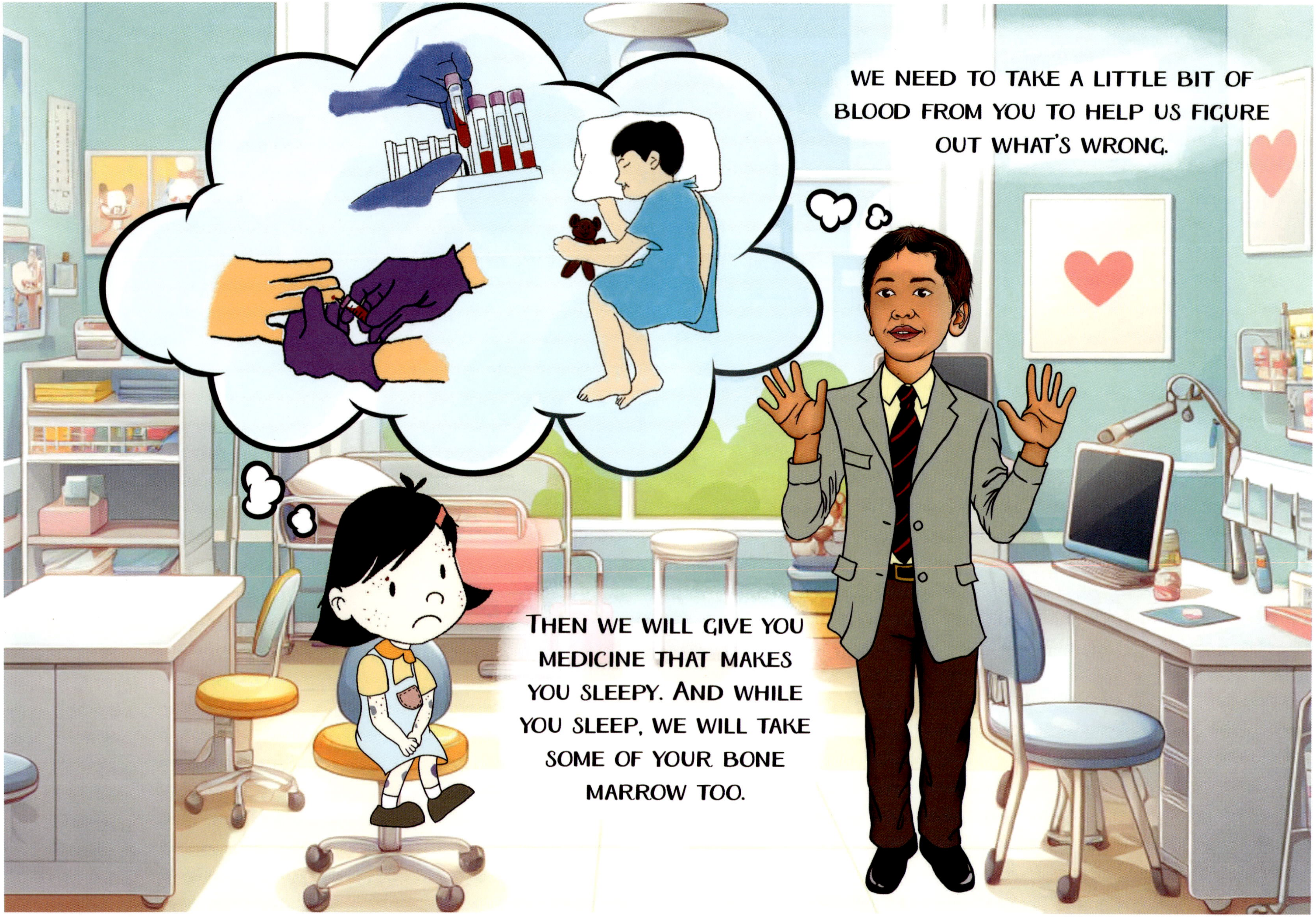
WE NEED TO TAKE A LITTLE BIT OF BLOOD FROM YOU TO HELP US FIGURE OUT WHAT'S WRONG.
THEN WE WILL GIVE YOU MEDICINE THAT MAKES YOU SLEEPY. AND WHILE YOU SLEEP, WE WILL TAKE SOME OF YOUR BONE MARROW TOO.

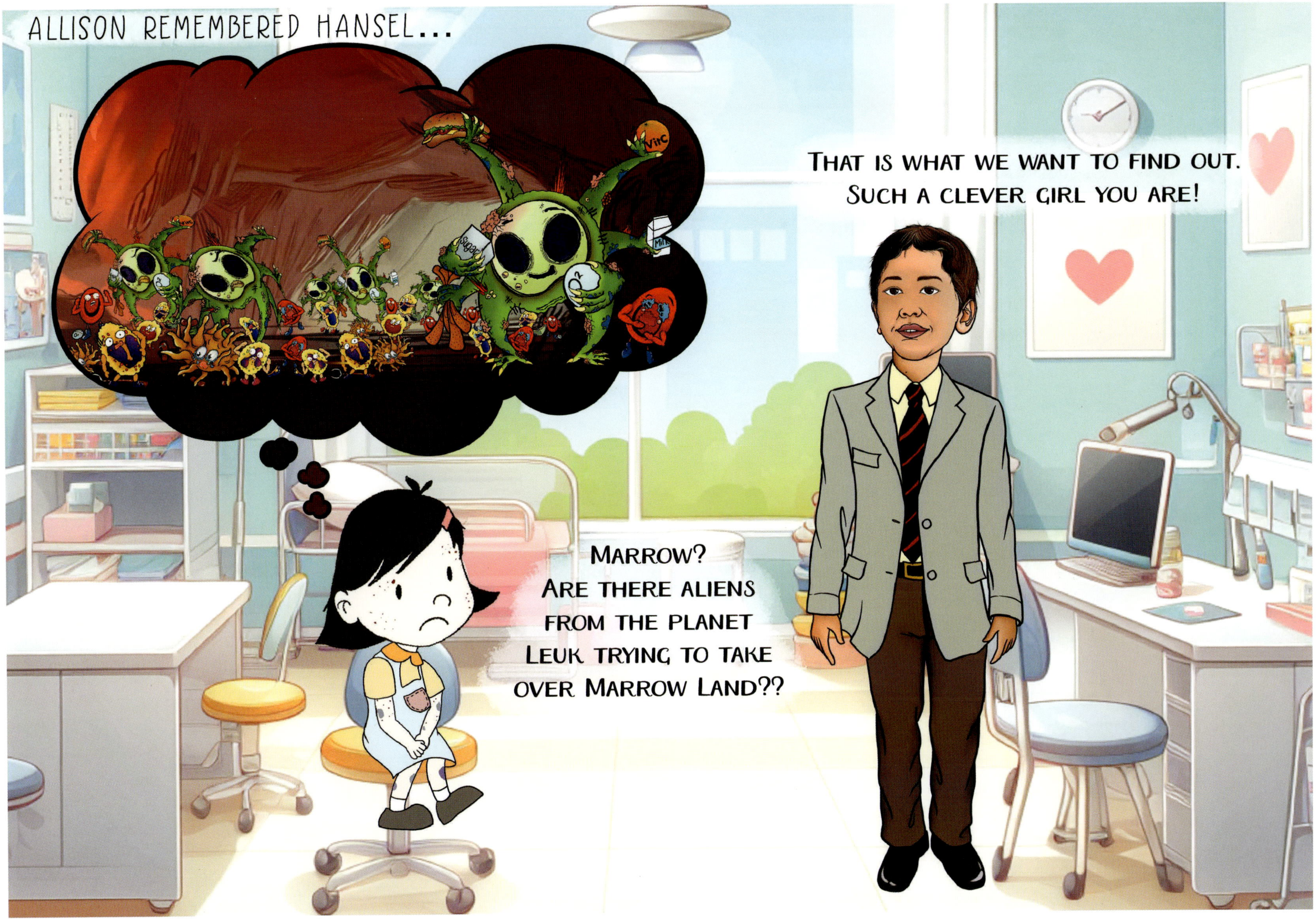
ALLISON REMEMBERED HANSEL...
MARROW? ARE THERE ALIENS FROM THE PLANET LEUK TRYING TO TAKE OVER MARROW LAND??
THAT IS WHAT WE WANT TO FIND OUT. SUCH A CLEVER GIRL YOU ARE!

BUT ALLISON BEGAN TO WORRY...

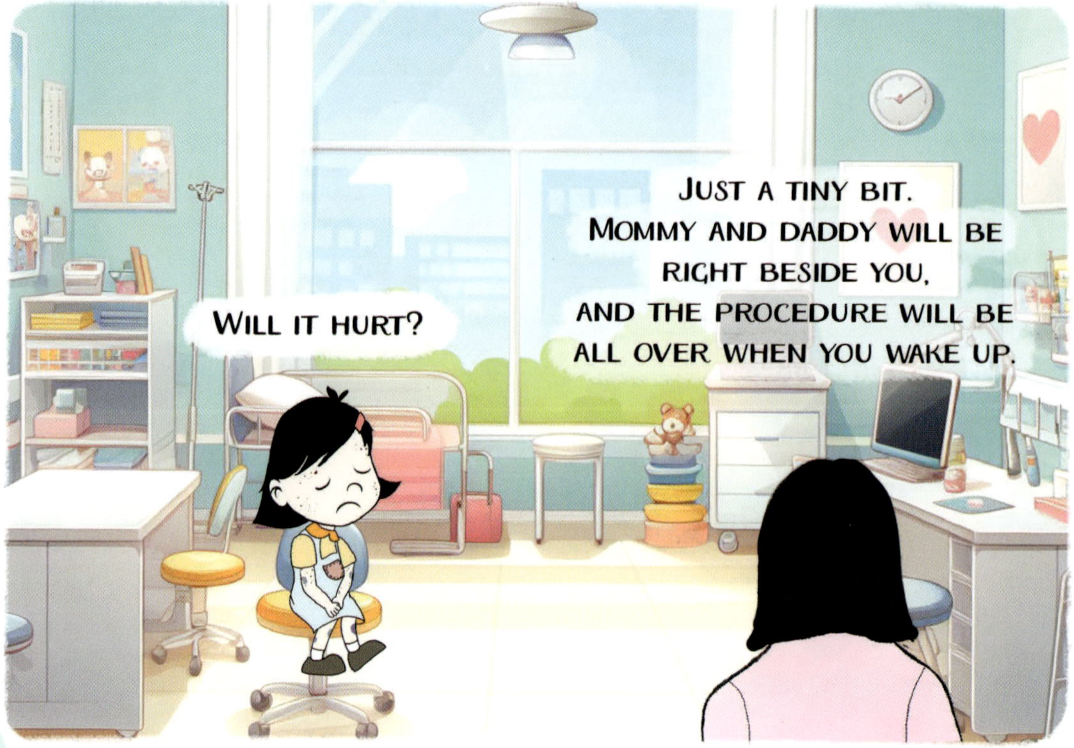
WILL IT HURT?
JUST A TINY BIT.
MOMMY AND DADDY WILL BE
RIGHT BESIDE YOU,
AND THE PROCEDURE WILL BE
ALL OVER WHEN YOU WAKE UP.

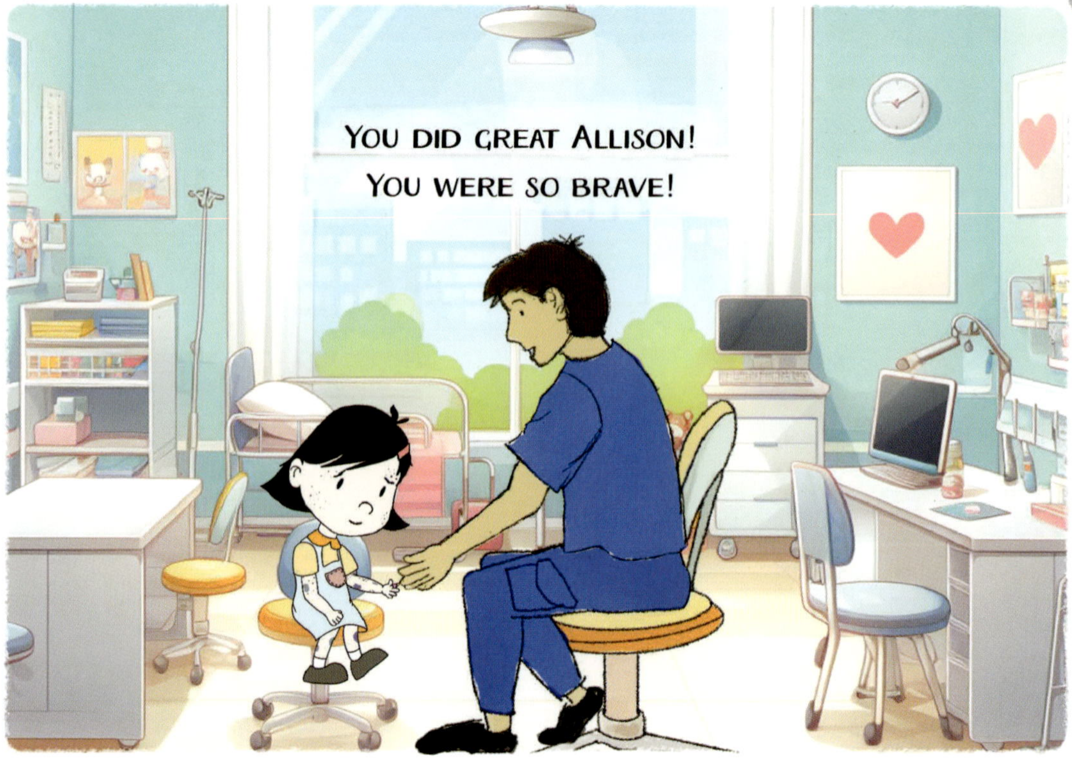
YOU DID GREAT ALLISON!
YOU WERE SO BRAVE!

A NURSE CAME TO TAKE BLOOD FROM HER FINGER, AND ALLISON WAS SURPRISED THAT IT HURT ONLY A LITTLE BIT, AND JUST FOR A LITTLE WHILE!

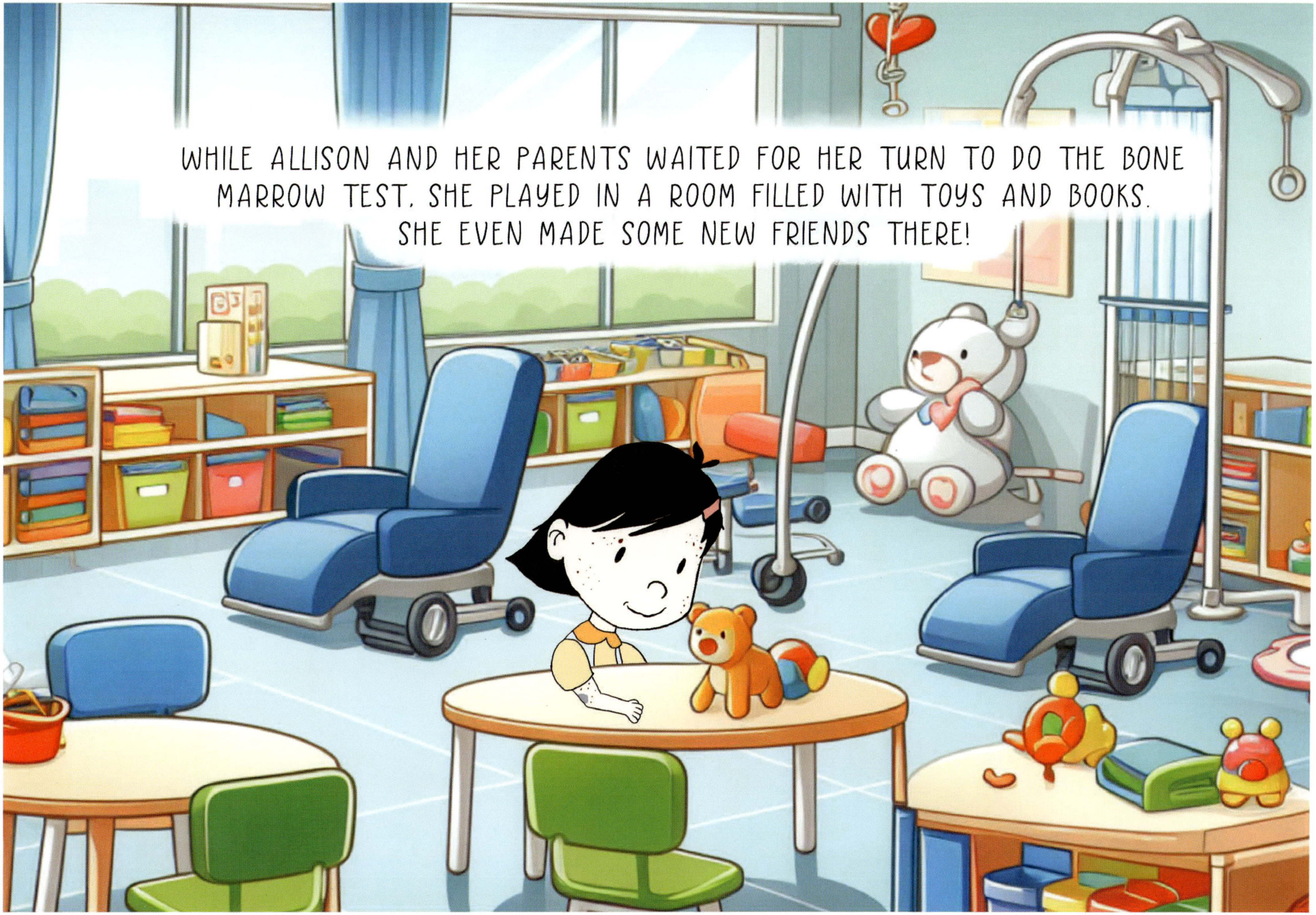

WHILE ALLISON AND HER PARENTS WAITED FOR HER TURN TO DO THE BONE MARROW TEST, SHE PLAYED IN A ROOM FILLED WITH TOYS AND BOOKS. SHE EVEN MADE SOME NEW FRIENDS THERE!

AFTER THE PROCEDURE...

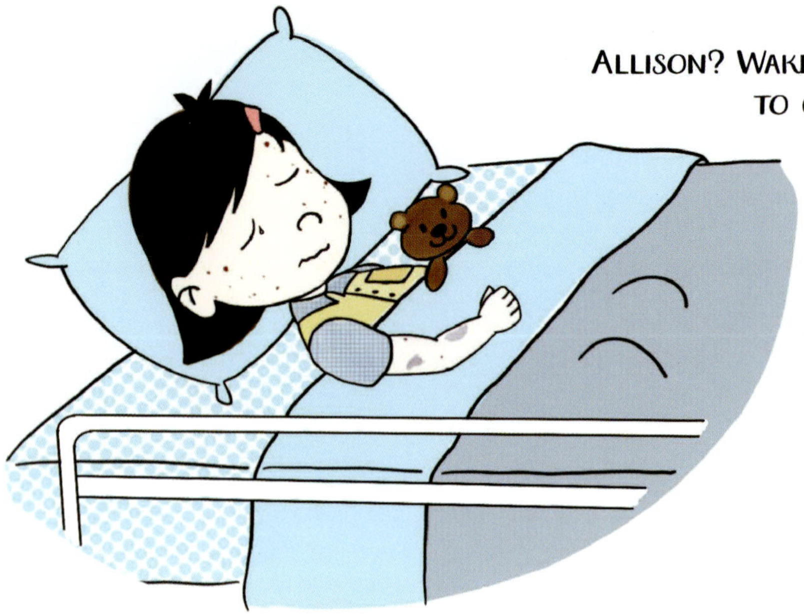
ALLISON? WAKE UP DEAR. IT'S TIME TO GO HOME.

THAT NIGHT, ALLISON HAD ANOTHER STRANGE DREAM.

SHE FOUND HERSELF BACK IN MARROW LAND.

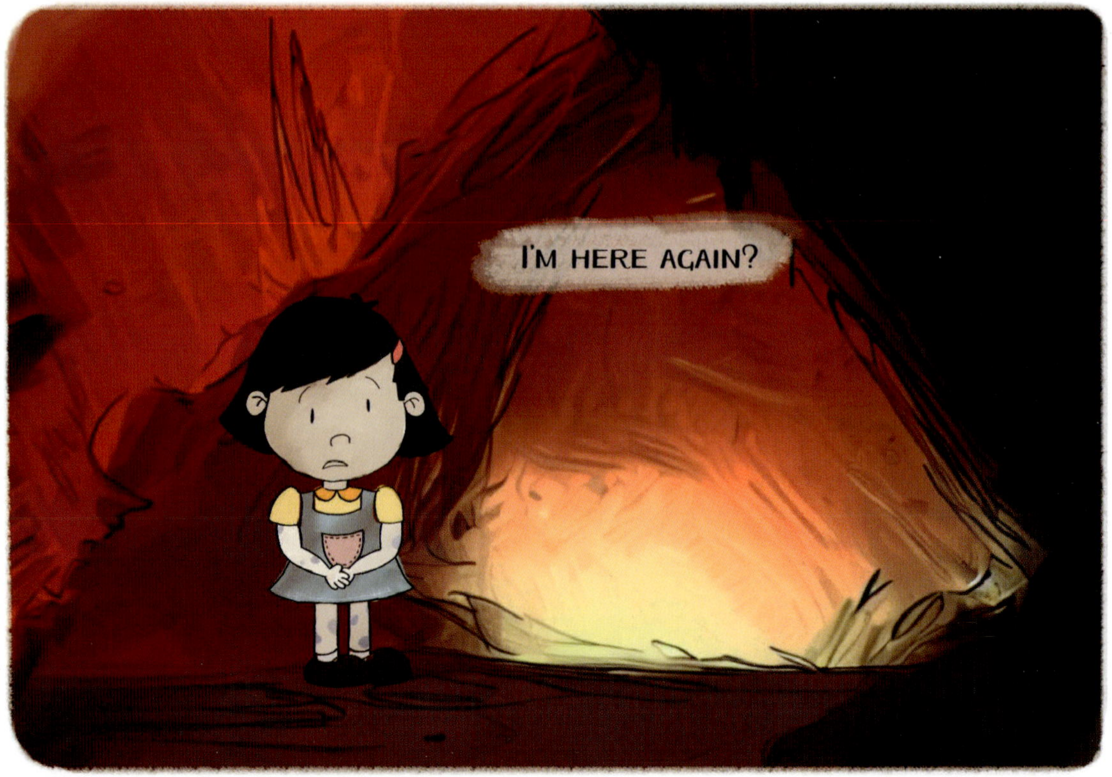
I'M HERE AGAIN?

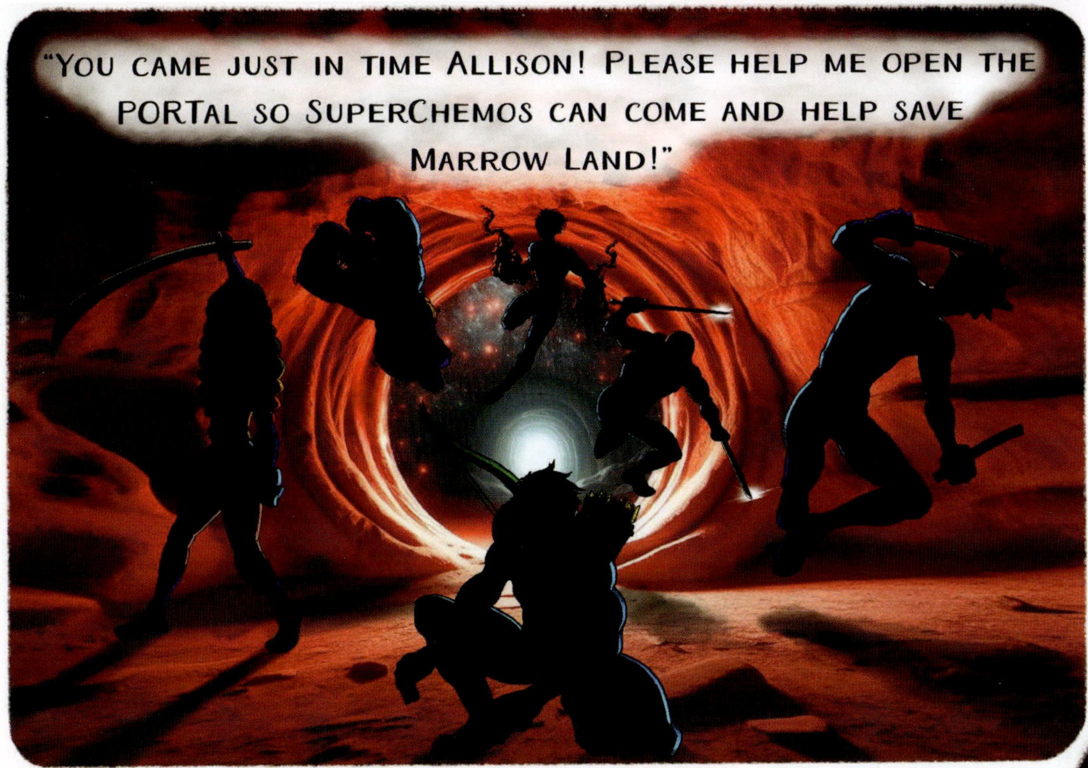
"You came just in time Allison! Please help me open the PORTal so SuperChemos can come and help save Marrow Land!"

"What's a PORTal?"

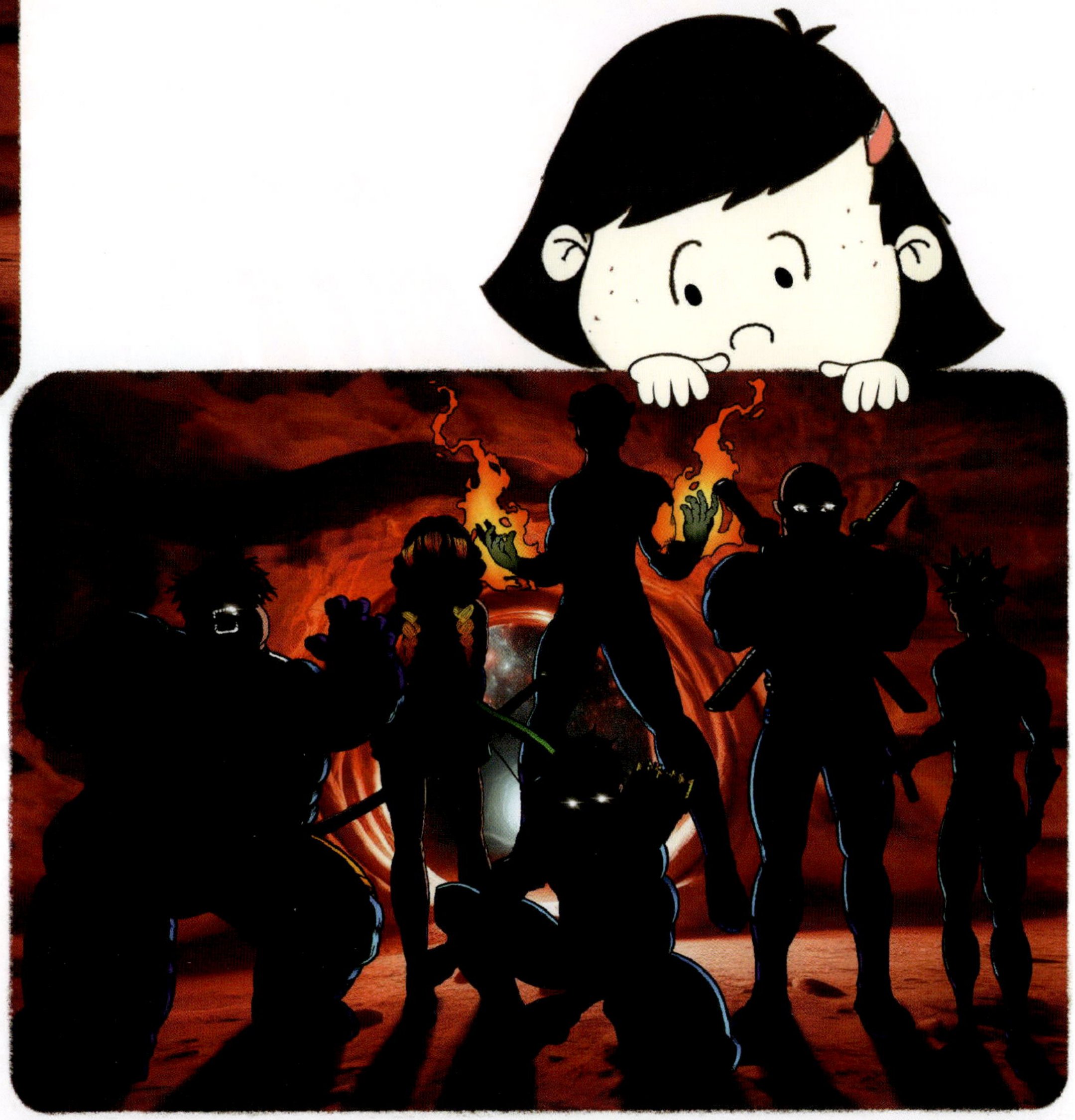

"It's the fastest and safest way SuperChemos can enter Marrow Land!"

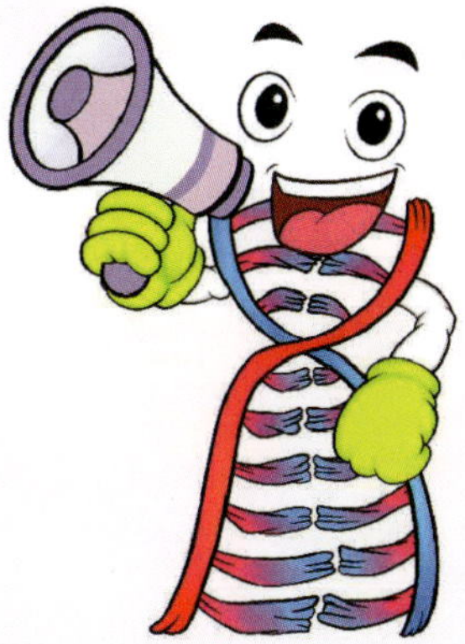

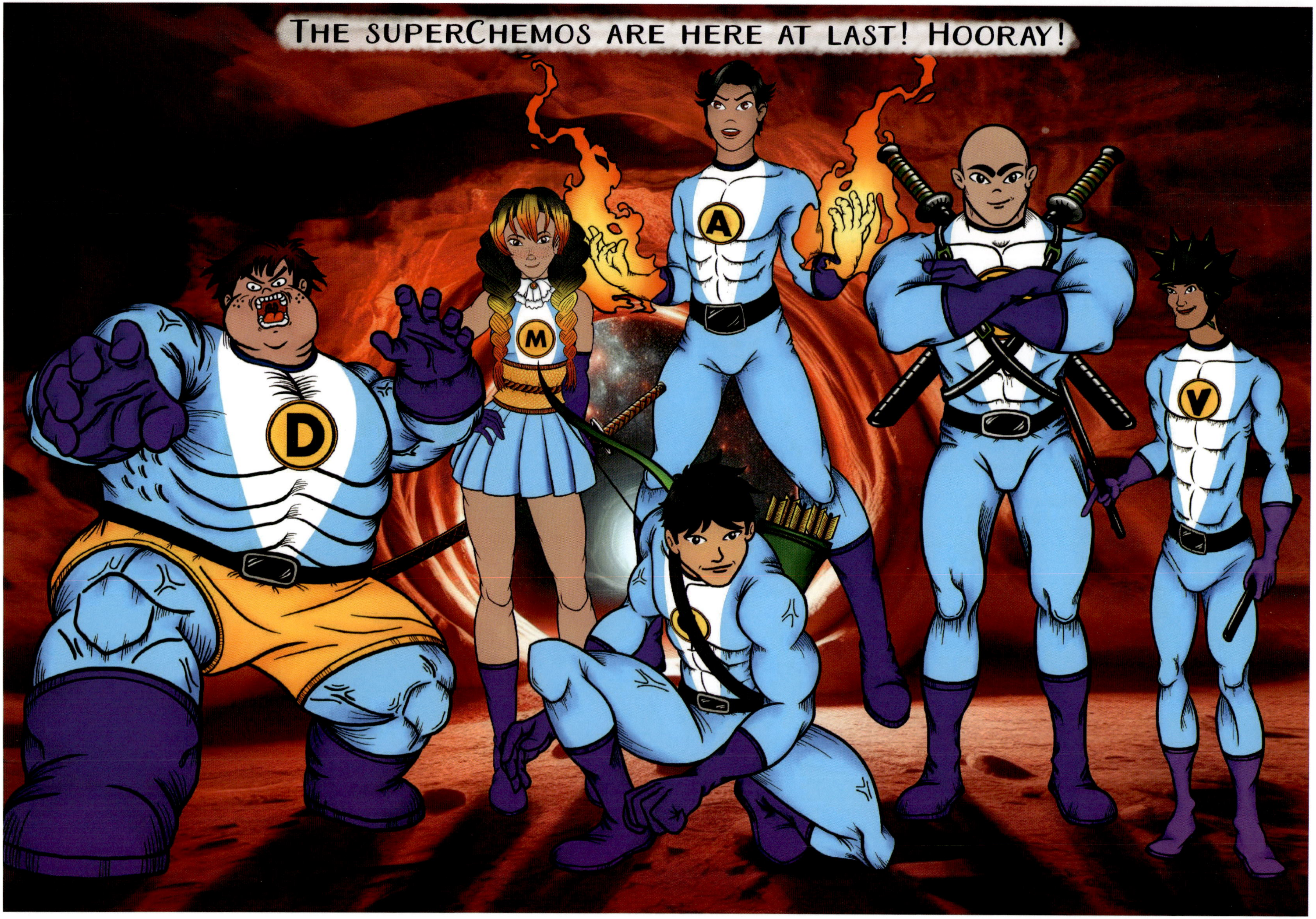
THE SUPERCHEMOS ARE HERE AT LAST! HOORAY!

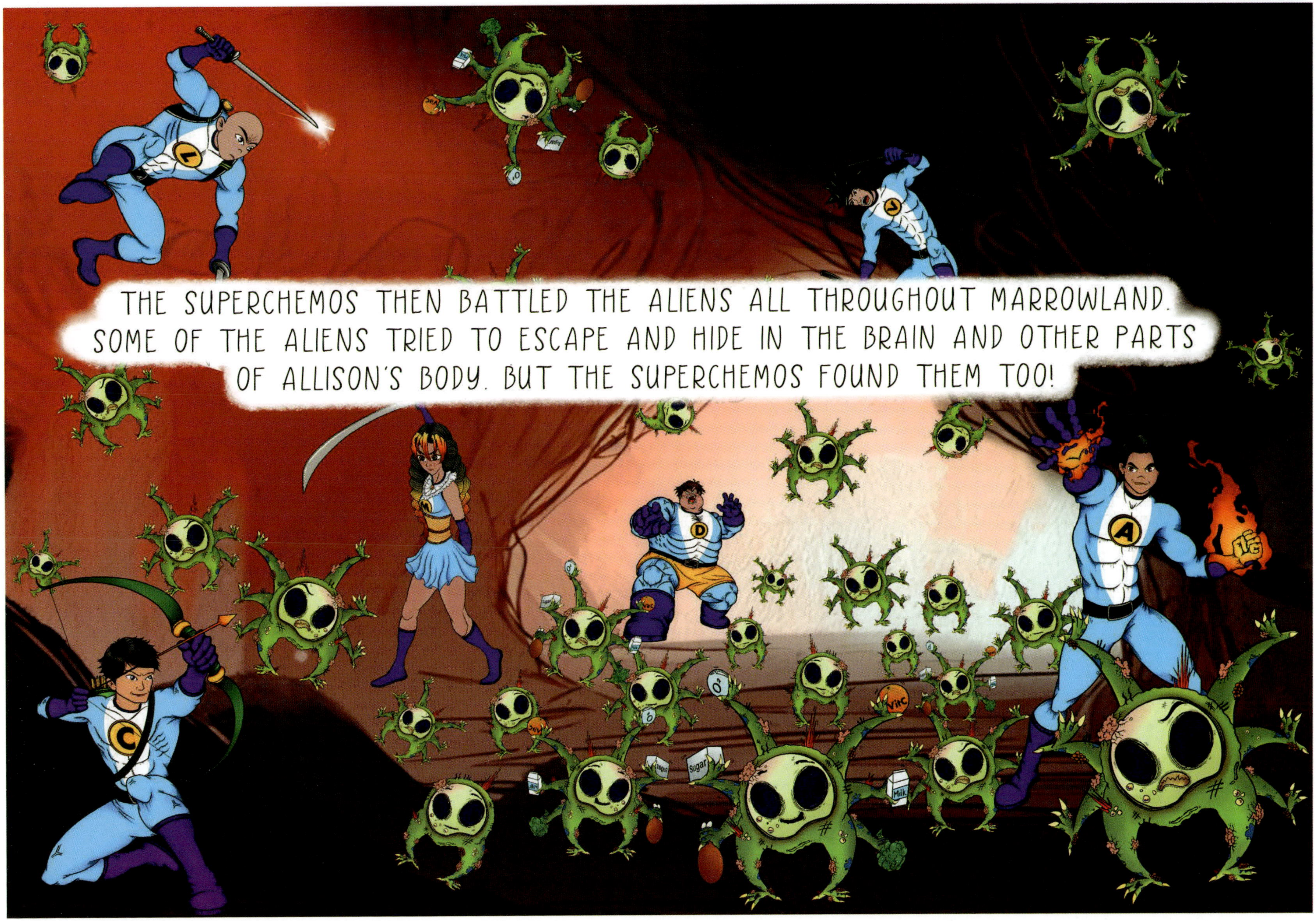
THE SUPERCHEMOS THEN BATTLED THE ALIENS ALL THROUGHOUT MARROWLAND. SOME OF THE ALIENS TRIED TO ESCAPE AND HIDE IN THE BRAIN AND OTHER PARTS OF ALLISON'S BODY. BUT THE SUPERCHEMOS FOUND THEM TOO!

ALLISON WOKE UP TO THE SOUND OF HER MOM TALKING TO SOMEONE ON THE PHONE.

"ALLISON, THAT WAS THE HOSPITAL. WE NEED TO GO SO WE WON'T BE LATE FOR OUR APPOINTMENT WITH DR ANSEL."

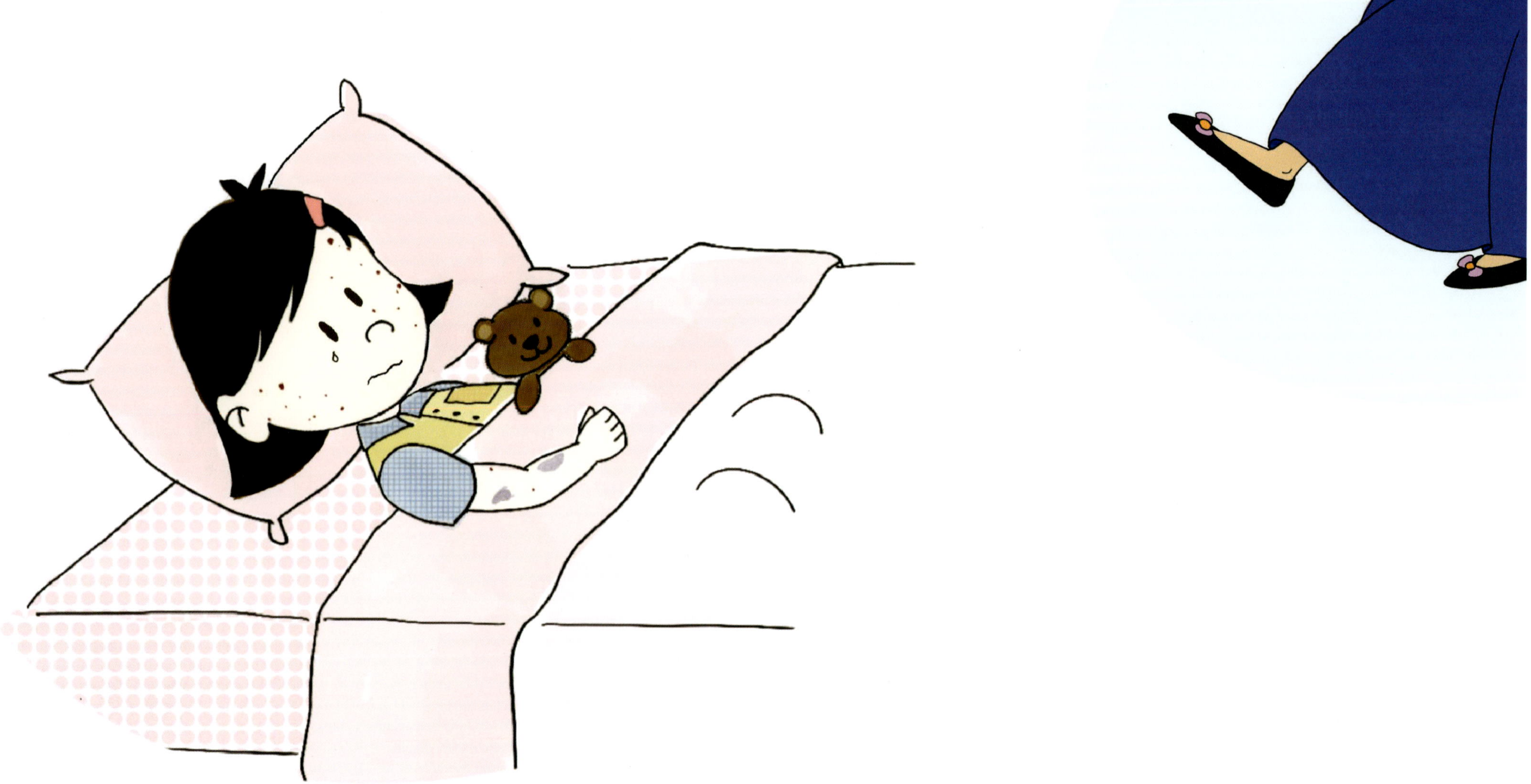

AT THE HOSPITAL, DR ANSEL EXPLAINED THE RESULTS OF ALLISON'S BONE MARROW TEST.

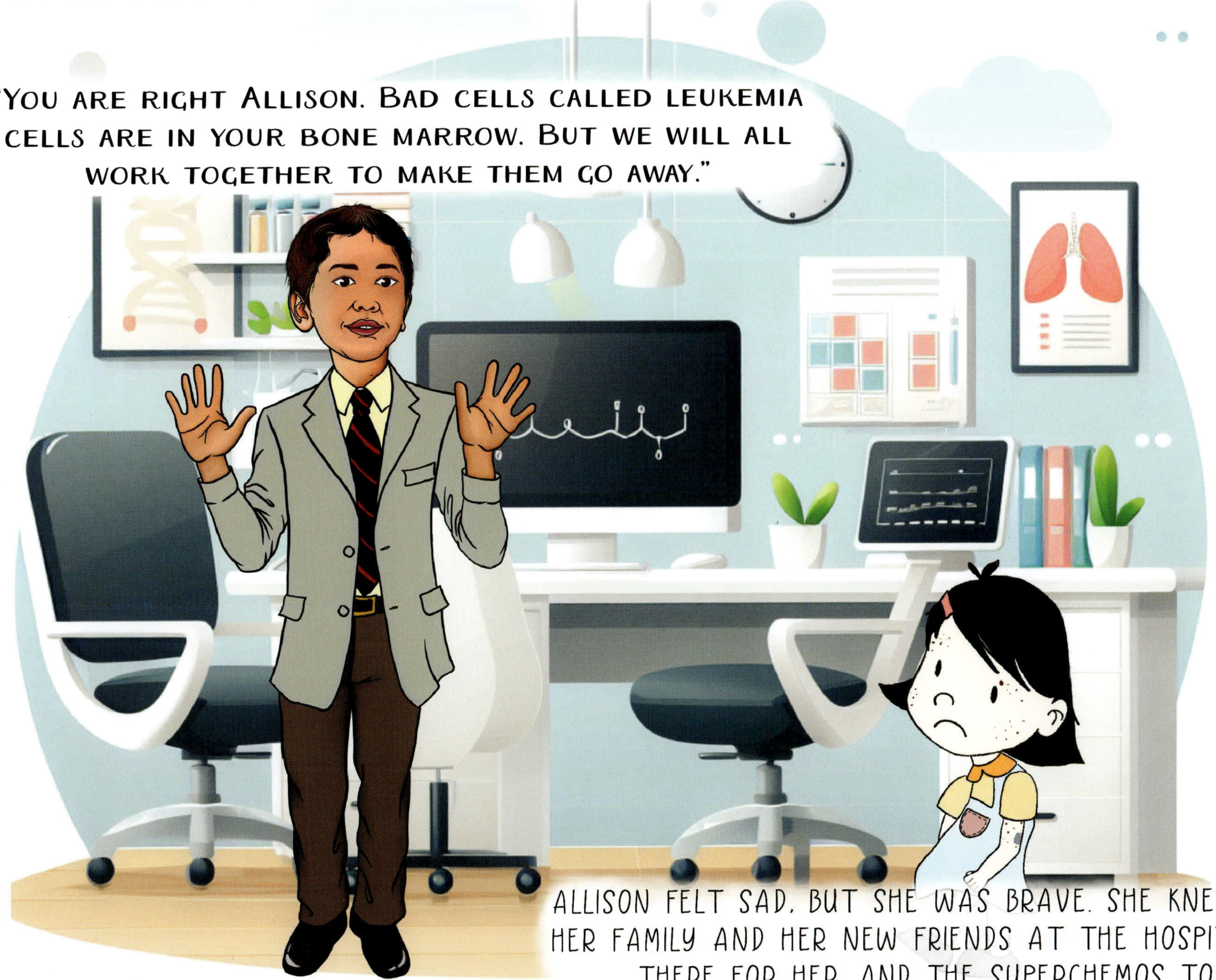
"YOU ARE RIGHT ALLISON. BAD CELLS CALLED LEUKEMIA CELLS ARE IN YOUR BONE MARROW. BUT WE WILL ALL WORK TOGETHER TO MAKE THEM GO AWAY."

ALLISON FELT SAD, BUT SHE WAS BRAVE. SHE KNEW THAT HER FAMILY AND HER NEW FRIENDS AT THE HOSPITAL ARE THERE FOR HER, AND THE SUPERCHEMOS TOO!

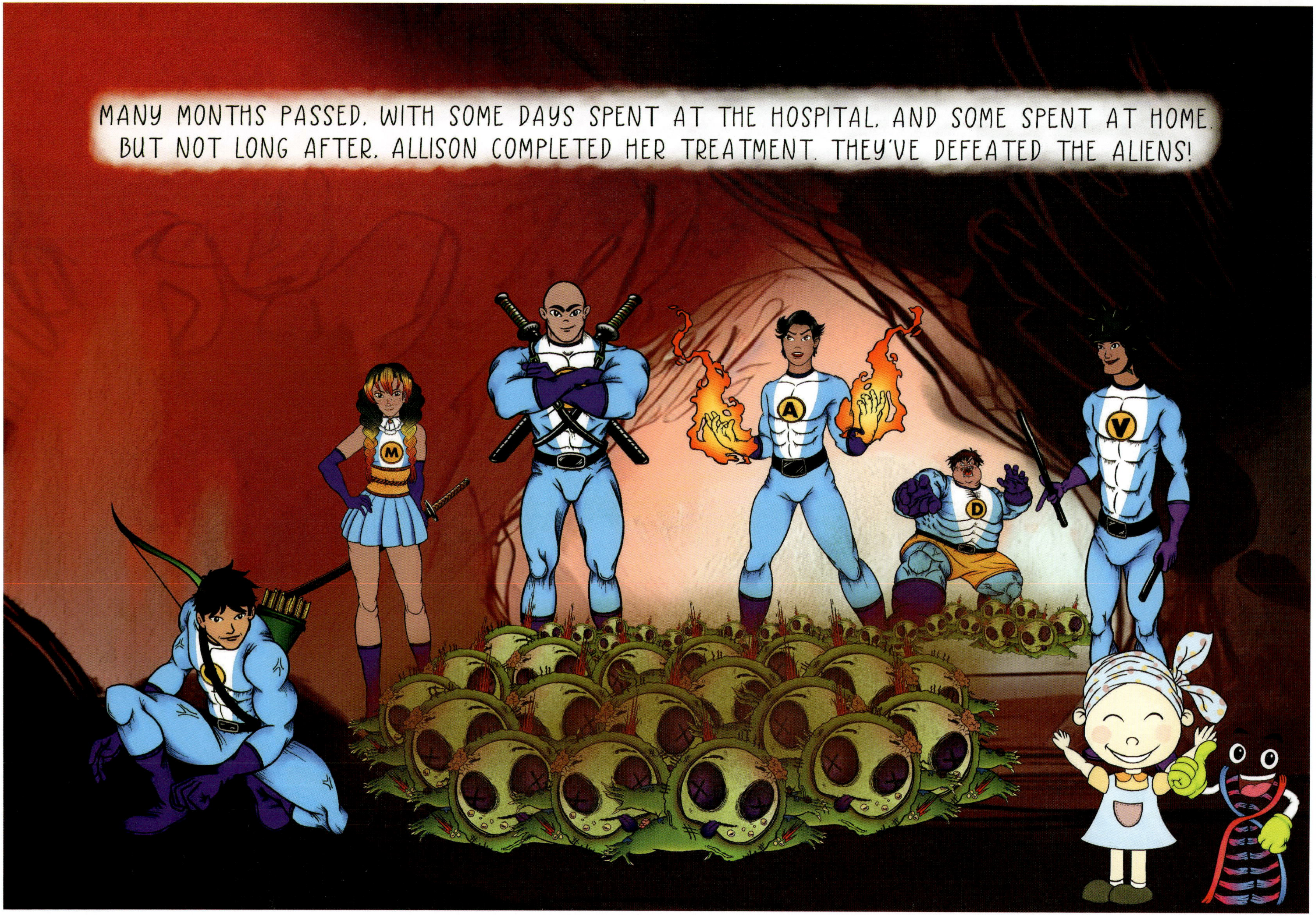
MANY MONTHS PASSED, WITH SOME DAYS SPENT AT THE HOSPITAL, AND SOME SPENT AT HOME. BUT NOT LONG AFTER, ALLISON COMPLETED HER TREATMENT. THEY'VE DEFEATED THE ALIENS!
M
A
D
V

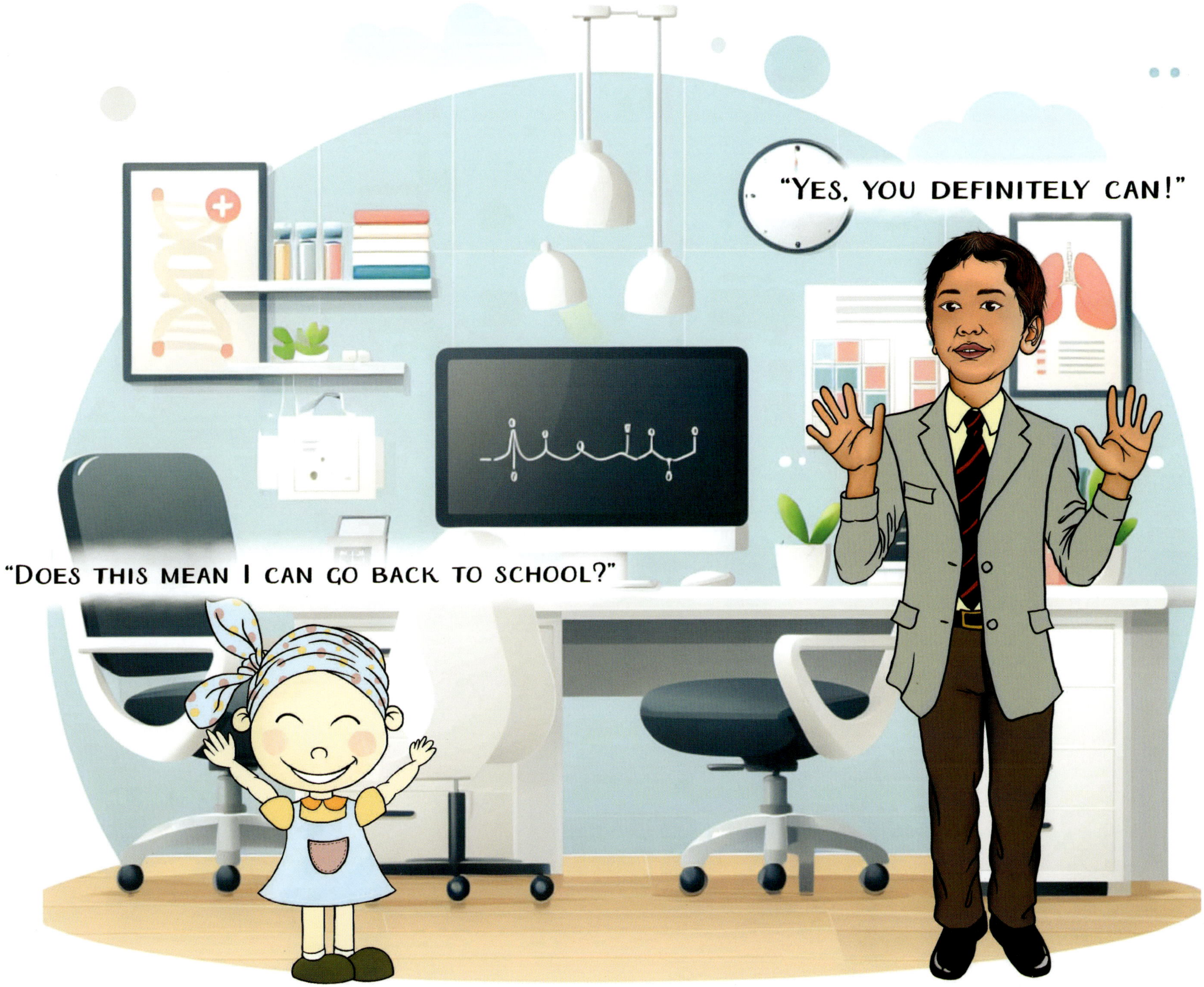
"YES, YOU DEFINITELY CAN!"
"DOES THIS MEAN I CAN GO BACK TO SCHOOL?"

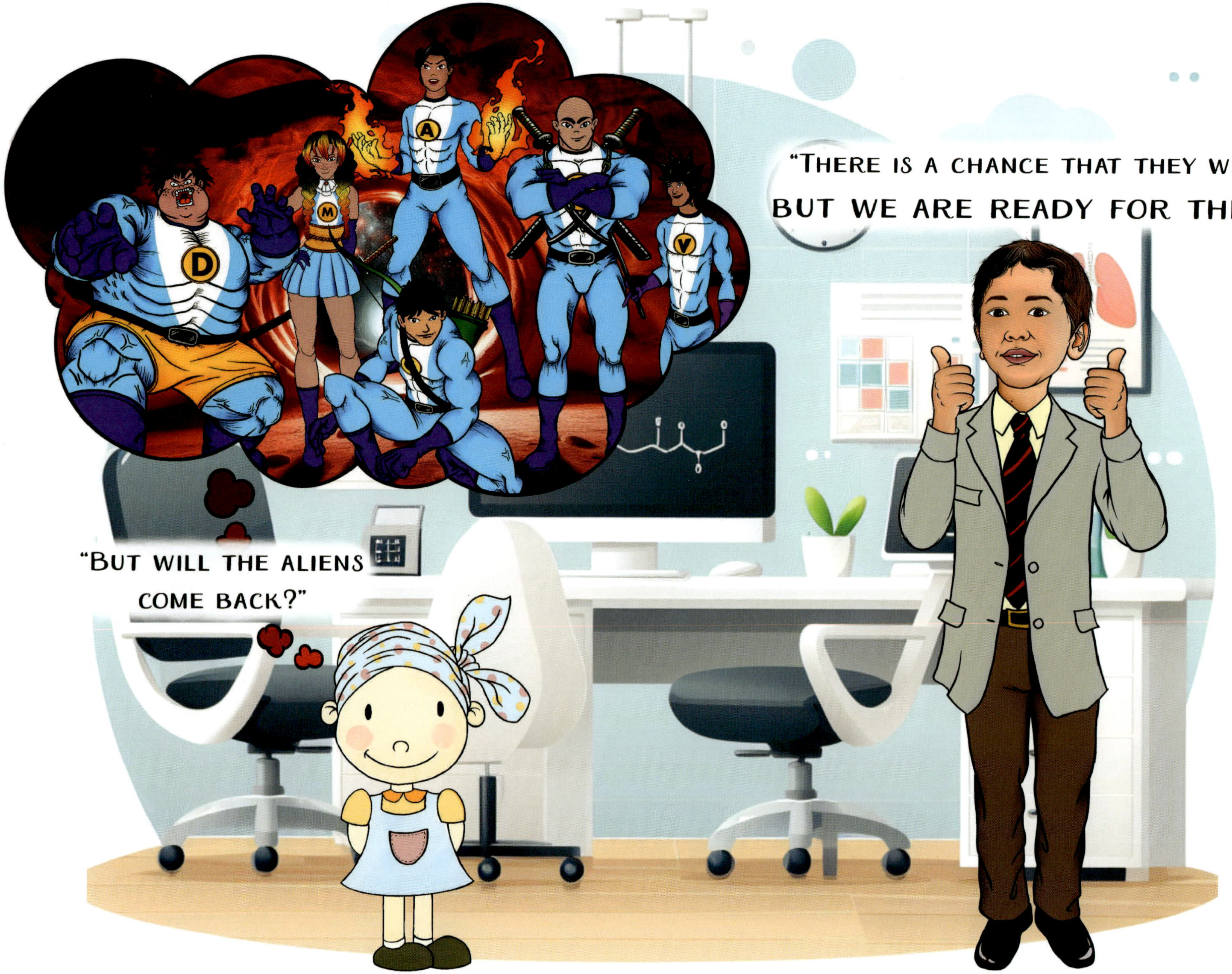

"BUT WILL THE ALIENS COME BACK?"
"THERE IS A CHANCE THAT THEY WILL, BUT WE ARE READY FOR THEM."

THE END

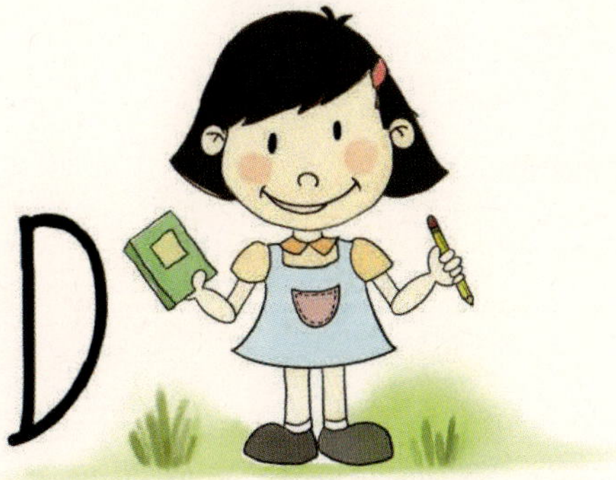